THE
SEAWEED
BEAUTY
GUIDE

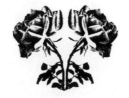

THE SEAWEED BEAUTY GUIDE

Simply Natural!

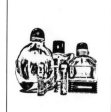 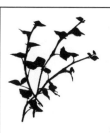  

Luxurious, Homemade,
Ph-balanced Skin-Care

CLAYTEN TYLOR

Tylor, Clayten

The Seaweed Beauty Guide:
Simply Natural!
Luxurious, Homemade, Ph-balanced Skin-Care.
Published 2009 by Lulu.com
Second Edition

ISBN 978-0-557-23782-1

Beauty / Seaweed (Marine Algae) / Herbs

**Copyright © 2009
by Clayten Tylor.**

Some sections of this book previously appeared in the author's other published book *The Seaweed Jelly-Diet Cookbook Guide (2008)*.

All rights reserved.

No portion of this book except for brief review, may be reproduced, stored in a retrieval system, or transmitted in any form or by any means – electronic, mechanical, photocopying, recording, or otherwise - without the written permission of the publisher. For information contact the publisher: Lulu.com

The information in this book is true and complete to the best of our knowledge. All recommendations are made without guarantee on the part of the author or publisher. The author and publisher disclaim any liability in connection with the use of this information.

Cover photos,
pictures and book design by Clayten Tylor

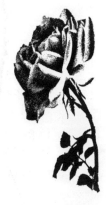
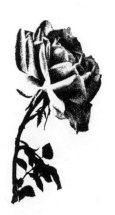

TABLE OF CONTENTS

Preface... Page Viii

INTRODUCTION - *1*
How This Book Came About .. .. Page 1
About The Recipes: .... Page 2

CHAPTER ONE: SEAWEED PREPARATION - *3*
About Seaweed Extracts... Page 5
About Brown Seaweed.. Page 6
About Green & Red Seaweed..................................... Page 7
Natural Seaweed Jells... Page 8
    Making The Scented Serum Recipe......................... Page 9
    Making The Scented Jelly Recipe............................ Page 10
    Making The Scented Paste Recipe.......................... Page 11
    Herbal Distillation Process.......................................Page 12

CHAPTER TWO: FACE & BODY SCRUBS - *13*
About The Face & Body Scrubs................................. Page 15
    Salt Scrub.. Page 16
    Clay Scrub... Page 17
    Oatmeal Scrub.. Page 18
    Milk & Honey Peeling Scrub.................................... Page 19
    Exfoliating Body Scrub.. Page 20

CHAPTER THREE: SKIN CARE - *21*
About The Skin Care Recipe....................................... Page 23
    Moisturizing Jelly... Page 24
    Moisturizing Body Soap... Page 25
    Astringent Jelly.. Page 26
    Splash Toner Rinse... Page 27
    Lotus-root Under-eye Salve..................................... Page 28
    Massage Oil.. Page 29
    Elbows & Knees : Intensive Moisturizer................... Page 30

CHAPTER FOUR: SUN CARE - *31*

About The Sun Care Jelly.. Page 33
    Suntan Lotion.. Page 34
    Sunburn Lotion... Page 35
    After-Sun Lotion... Page 36
    Self-tanning Bronze Lotion.. Page 37
    Joy Jelly.. Page 38

CHAPTER FIVE: BATH & SHOWER - *39*

About The Bath & Shower Recipes... Page 41
    Natural Bath Sachets... Page 42
    Hand & Body Soap.. Page 43
    Baby Powder Deodorant Jelly... Page 44
    Moisturizing Hair Rinse.. Page 45
    Tooth Paste Polish... Page 46

CHAPTER SIX: SPA TREATMENTS - *47*

About: Spa Treatments.. Page 49
    Reformation Clay Facial Mask... Page 50
    Moisturizing Detox Bath... Page 51
    Face & Body Polish... Page 52
    Wrinkle Reducing Body Treatment.. Page 53
    Neutralizing Red Seaweed Treatment..................................... Page 53

CHAPTER SEVEN: HERBAL BEAUTY TREATMENTS - *55*

Herbal Beauty Treatments.. Page 57
Seven Principles of Cellular Regeneration..................................... Page 58
Beauty Balancing Treatments... Page 59

CHAPTER EIGHT: HOMEOPATHIC HEALING - *75*

Homeopathic Energy Medicine: Color Therapy.............................. Page 77
Energy Medicine Skin Area Treatments... Page 78
Homeopathic Cell Salt Tonic... Page 79

BIBLIOGRAPHY - *81*
HERB CHARTS: LATIN NAMES - *85*
PLANETARY HOUR RULER CHARTS - *87*
NUTRITIONAL CHARTS – *89*

PREFACE

Where I Am Coming From

We have all experienced the slimy texture of seaweed while at the ocean beach, but how many of us have experienced first-hand the beautiful jelling compounds that seaweed has to offer when it is exposed to just fresh water.

I am not a scientist, and the recipes in this book have only been tested on my own skin. However, I have always been interested in testing and trying new things, especially subjects like metaphysics, ancient wisdom, and alchemy, subjects that test and try the assumptions we make about our self, and about the things of nature.

These subjects essentially teach the science of determining the inner nature of a thing, or a person, whether a personality flaw, or the benefits of a particular herb or treatment. It is the science of the body from the inside out, from a spiritual perspective, such as how the blood draws into itself the nutrients it needs, or how the brain restricts only the purer blood by its rate of contraction, and how these natural rhythms may be better regulated.

All of these subjects deal with understanding and initiating the seven creative principles of regeneration. From cellular regeneration used in spiritual healing, to spiritual regeneration, which transfers the sense of self, from being a 'body,' to being 'spirit'. These inner processes only need to be acknowledged and encouraged to perform their work more effectively.

Nevertheless, even when we understand how the mind may become the instrument for change - we still age, get ugly, and die. But, we do not have to feel ugly while we age. And that is the key to outer beauty - inner beauty!

However, no matter how strong our sense of inner beauty is, it cannot radiate through a beauty product that you can feel on your skin. If you can feel your beauty product on your skin then it is really a cosmetic. You should not be able to feel where your skin ends, and the atmosphere begins, a pH-balanced connection to the universe.

This is where that slimy seaweed comes in, for it is soothing to open sores, chapped skin, cuts, burns, and itchy skin. Although this book uses essentially just one seaweed compound, each chapter is set up to explain how it can be used in a variety of different ways, as a binder, a stabilizer, an emollient, or a creaming agent, to combine with other ingredients to help repair and regenerate the skin.

Combining the luxurious gelling compounds of seaweed, with a simple 'no-fuss, no-muss', daily skin-care regime, you too can create your own non-toxic, natural, pH-balanced skin care products that are fun to make, and safe enough for the whole family to use daily.

In addition, just like with the study of metaphysics, if you do not actually do any of the 'inner work' on your personality - and in this case - if you do not actually apply any of these recipes - it will all remain an intellectual concept, and you will never really know how easy it is to coax such a luxurious product, from such a slimy substance.

Enjoy!

INTRODUCTION

How this Book Came About

The interest in writing this book was never from the aspect of using seaweed for skin care. In fact my skin, seldom, if ever, had seen a moisturizer or a body lotion in its entire life. Now I understand why, it was because I had never found anything which I could put on my skin that felt good - until now.

This book began after publishing the first book called 'The Seaweed Jelly-Diet Cookbook Guide', which was about the discoveries while experimenting with seaweed as food. In which I continually found myself with several batches of seaweed being prepared, and nothing to do with them.

One day, after being at the beach I got sun burnt badly on the chest, and was trying to find a way to apply apple-cider vinegar, to relieve the pain and assist with the healing. Instead of soaking paper towels and laying them on the chest, I decided to mix apple-cider vinegar with some of the clear seaweed jelly that was being prepared. It was such a relief, that the Seaweed Beauty Guide began to emerge.

I then started to add the seaweed jelly to other skin care products, and was impressed with the improved moisturizing effects. I tried other treatments such as the clay facial, a treatment that can be very messy and extremely drying. Amazingly, the seaweed not only held the clay together, but also added a rich moisturizing effect, something I had not ever experienced in conjunction with clay – it was incredible!

As I refined the seaweed recipes, the odor became more tolerable, and the consistency more creamy, and it could then be worn throughout the day without being noticed. This expanded its uses into applications such as the herbal treatments, which required it to be not only protective and moisturizing, but also invisible.

Many times while writing the book I got discouraged thinking this book did not really say anything new, and then I would discover another use, like the Baby-Powder Deodorant, so simple, yet effective, and I would continue. The only thing that might be new is the fact that I am not going to make a seaweed moisturizer, add chemicals, and sell it to you for a thousand dollars an ounce. Instead, anyone, rich or poor, can now have the finest beauty products that nature can provide.

I hope you enjoy the simplicity of these techniques, and are able to carry them forward by adding your own combinations to make your own luxuriant skin-care products. Then one day you might even want to try eating Seaweed, as described in the Seaweed Jelly-Diet Cookbook Guide. Remember, you only have to 'try it' to believe.

ABOUT THE RECIPES

Seaweed Skin-Care

Seaweed 'Jelly' is the term I use to distinguish it from seaweed 'Gels' and 'extracts' that have been processed using chemicals. Those chemically extracted gels are in every beauty product that has ever touched your skin. In fact, if the product felt luxurious and creamy, it probably had some seaweed extract in it to make it feel that way. However, the recipes in this book use only natural seaweed jelly - same creamy texture without the chemicals.

Some of the recipes for the skin treatments are washed-off immediately, while others such as herbal treatments are gentle enough to leave on your skin all day and night. None of the recipes are harsh enough to hurt your skin; all of them are luxurious enough to want to leave them on all the time, you decide. In addition, if you want these recipes to pass the 'kiss test', you might want to add your favorite flower essence or perfume.

In addition, most of these recipes are for a single application, enough for just the face, and because they do not contain preservatives or alcohol, would easily spoil unless kept refrigerated. Therefore, if you want to make these recipes in larger quantities, you will need to add your own preservative.

If you just want to add some seaweed to your store-bought skin-care products such as your liquid hand soap or shower gel, then no additional preservative is required. This is an excellent way to benefit from seaweed jells without any changes to your skin care routine. Just wash and moisturize at the same time - great for getting your whole family's skin soft without chemicals.

In addition, the three preparation techniques used to make the seaweed Serum, Jelly, and Paste recipes use dried seaweed only. I tried using fresh seaweed, but the odor in the finished product was far too strong. (Although the fact that the fresh seaweed had been washed-up on to the beach, and I had no idea where its actual source was from, which could have accounted for the strong odor).

I still recommend that you start with the dried Kelp, so that you are not discouraged by the initial result. I think because the dried kelp holds less water, and that the odor must be in the water - therefore the less water (dried), the less smell.

I have also included some spiritual quotes, by Emanuel Swedenborg. These quotes explain the 'inner nature' of an ingredient through spiritual correspondence. It gives a clue as to what to expect from mixing different herbs and ingredients. Spiritual quotes lift the mind to an 'ah-ha' moment, and I will attempt to decipher the more complicated ones, in the hope that you can appreciate the true spiritual perspective of 'really natural' beauty products.

CHAPTER ONE: SEAWEED PREPARATION

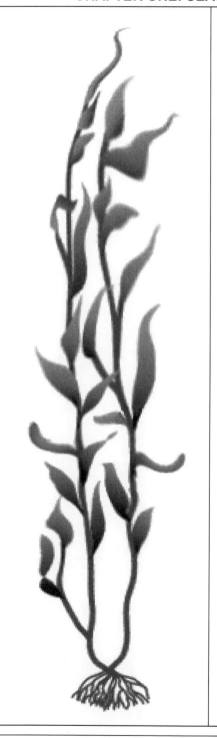

"In the universal heaven, every individual is a center of the blessedness and happiness of all, and all together are the center of the blessedness and happiness of each individual."

(Swedenborg A.C. 2872)

ABOUT SEAWEED EXTRACTS

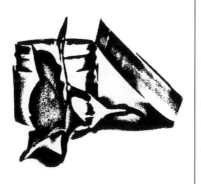

"The Divine cannot be appropriated to man as his own, but may be adjoined to him, and thereby appear as his own."

- Swedenborg. D.P. 285

Seaweed - The World's Most Luxurious Gels

Seaweed contains the world's most luxurious gelling compounds, used in almost every beauty product. In fact, seaweeds are the only natural plant source for gelling and emulsifying agents.

The patents for the extraction process date back to 1922, and read like alchemical doctrine, probably to disguise the simplicity of the process, which uses chemicals such as hydrochloric acid and bleach to clean and remove the gels.

The process requires approval by the food and drug administration, which classifies it as an extract, yet does not require these chemicals to be included on the ingredient list. The chemicals are only used to simplify the separation of the liquid gels from the solid matter - which can be done without chemicals or preservatives, if done in small amounts, as explained in this book.

Seaweed Extracts & Chemicals

If you have skin sensitivities, it is time to kick the seaweed extracts habit, and start using unprocessed seaweed jelly.

The seaweed gels are known as Algal polysaccharides, which are gelatinous substances, mucilaginous in nature, and depending on the chemicals used, and the type of seaweed, these gels are known by many other names such as Aginic acid, agar, carrageenin, laminarin, fucoidin, galactans, xylems, and mannans.

These seaweed extracts are used as emulsifiers, stabilizers, and thickeners, in most cosmetics, shampoos, shaving creams, anti-bacterial gels and ointments. Therefore, unless your skin care product says just 'seaweed', it is actually an extract - and those chemicals are on your skin right now.

ABOUT BROWN SEAWEED

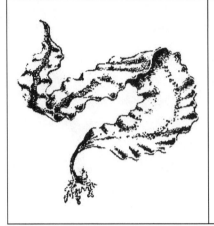

"Diaphanous forms transmit spiritual light, as crystal transmits natural."

- Swedenborg.- D.L.W. 245

About the Brown Seaweeds:

You can differentiate between the seaweed species by their color - red, brown, or green. The *brown* seaweed is used in all of these recipes because it contains the best gelling properties to bind the other ingredients.

In most of the recipes, I use brown seaweed (kelp) from Korea. However, it is better to look for kelp in general, locally and imported, then it is to attempt to find a specific species, which might not be available in your area.

All of the seaweeds are rich in vitamins A, B-1, B-2, B-6, C, Folic Acid, and Niacin, as well as contain 60 trace elements, B-12, vitamins E and K, and over 60 minerals, especially potassium, calcium, iodine, magnesium, phosphorus, iron, zinc, and manganese. (See Nutritional Chart).

Each species also has a Latin name, and I have included a list of the more common brown seaweeds. I have highlighted the large brown kelp, which might help you determine your local variety of kelp more easily.

LATIN NAMES OF SOME BROWN SEAWEEDS ALSO KNOWN AS PHAEOPHYTA		
Alaria Esculenta	Cystoseira usneoides	**Laminaria digitata**
Ascophyllum nodosum	Dictyopteris membranacea	**Laminaria japonica**
Bifurcaria bifurcata	Dictyota dichotoma	**Laminaria longicruris**
Carpomitra costata	Fucus spiralis	Padina pavonica
Cladostephus spongiosus	Fucus serratus	Pelvetia caniculata
Colpomenia peregrina	Fucus vesiculosus	Phyllariopsis purpurascens
Colpomenia sinuosa	Halidrys siliquosa	Saccorhiza polyschides
Cutleria multifida	Halopteris scoparia	Sargassum vulgare
Cystoseira abies-marina	Halopteris filicina	Sargassum muticum
Cystoseira compressa	**Laminaria agardhii**	Sporochnus pedunculatus
Cystoseira discors	**Laminaria saccharina**	Zonaria tournefortii

ABOUT GREEN & RED SEAWEED

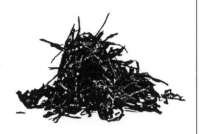

Dried Wakame Seaweed

"In every vegetable there is contained a use, a spiritual use in the spiritual world, and a spiritual and also a natural use in the natural world."

- Swedenborg. A.E. 1214

About the Green & Red Seaweeds

The Green and Red Seaweed species are used for the Spa treatments only, and chosen for their mineral content, and not their gelling properties. I have chosen only one variety of each, to demonstrate how they are used. A green Wakame seaweed from Japan, and a red Dulse seaweed from Canada. Again, choose a species of seaweed available in your area.

It is also very difficult to determine the type of seaweed from the packaging, let alone if it had been rinsed or not. Your best bet to choosing the correct species, is to familiarize yourself with the different local species.

Some Seaweed Preparation Tips:

The salt water used to dry seaweed kills all bacteria, and the only reason the dried seaweed needs rinsing is it reduce the salty odor. For the spa treatments, it is better to rinse the green and red seaweeds, because their odor can be too strong for an enjoyable spa treatment.

However, for the brown seaweed recipes, the gelling begins quicker, when the dried seaweed is not rinsed. Experiment by making a couple of small batches, a rinsed batch to wear in public, and a batch not rinsed, to where for private treatments. I have also included a distillation process (page 12) so that you can prepare the scented distilled water to use with the seaweed recipes.

In addition, the gelling stage begins quicker, 1-5 days, when the seaweed is soaked at room temperature, and 5-10 days if refrigerated. But it is a food and can also easily spoil, therefore, if you are in a hurry for your first batch, find a way to keep it just slightly cool, to speed up the jelling process.

NATURAL SEAWEED JELLS

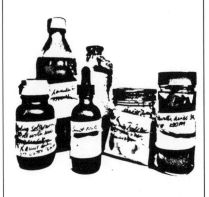

"Garden signifies the rational man destitute of rational truth."

- Swedenborg. A.C. 504

Types of Natural Seaweed Jells

The recipes in this book use three different seaweed jells. The first is a clear Serum made from dried Kelp, soaked in distilled scented water, and used in the skin and sun treatment recipes. The second is a pureed Jelly, also made from soaked Kelp, but used only in the Herbal Treatments recipes, in chapter five. The third is a pureed Seaweed Paste, made from either green or red seaweed, and used only in the Spa Treatments, in chapter seven.

1. Serum:

The Seaweed *Serum* is the name I use for the clear liquid egg-white jell that forms when seaweed encounters fresh water. It is the main ingredient used as the base in all of the recipes, and it may be made with distilled scented water. It binds and mixes the other ingredients into a smooth luxurious consistency - a kind of 'carrier' or 'transporter'. You may leave the *Serum*-based recipes on your skin day and night if needed, as used in the herbal skin treatments.

2. Jelly:

The Seaweed *Jelly* is soaked Kelp pureed in a blender to the consistency of a jelly. The additional liquid needed for the recipe, may be teas, distilled essences, or whatever liquid you desire. The *Jelly* is fine enough to wash off in the shower, therefore perfect for full body treatments.

3. Paste:

The seaweed *Paste* is made from the red or green seaweeds. The *Paste* has a longer drying time than the *Serum*, and is best for deep pore cleaning, spa treatments, and body wraps, or used to make poultices for the medicinal herbal treatments. It is perfect to blend with the *Serum* or *Jelly* for problem-skin intensive treatments.

MAKING THE SCENTED SERUM RECIPE

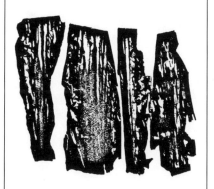

Dried Kelp

"All varieties of Sensation have reference to the sense of Touch."

- Swedenborg. 2528

1. Scented Seaweed Serum Recipe

This Seaweed Serum will keep for three weeks, if you keep everything clean in the beginning. Do not touch it with your fingers, be sure to cut it with clean scissors. Soak it in a clean glass or stainless steel container that has a pour spout, so that it is easier to pour. It freezes and thaws flawlessly.

- *1 Oz. dried brown Kelp Seaweed*
- *One Cup (250 ml) Distilled Scented Water*

Cut or break the dried Kelp into small equal pieces, for it lies flat, and then needs less water to cover. Put the dried kelp in a narrow container or jar. Press the dried seaweed down, and add just enough distilled scented water (as described in the following distillation recipe) to cover the seaweed. Soak for 24 hours covered at a cool temperature, stirring or shaking every few hours to keep the top moist, topping up with a little more water, only if needed, as the seaweed expands.

Refrigerate. When the *Serum* begins to thicken in 1-5 days, you can start to use it for your beauty treatments. However, keep refrigerated and do not add more water, otherwise it will be too thin.

Optional Rinsing:

For a less smelly serum, rinse the dried kelp quickly in *cold* water, but drain within a few seconds, before the gelling begins. Or, rinse it in the jar with fresh water - shake, and discard the rinsing water, immediately.

MAKING THE SCENTED JELLY RECIPE	
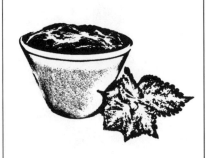	*"Affection, or love, is what constitutes the life of every person: for whatever the affection is, such is the whole man."* – Swedenborg. A.C. 288

2. Scented Seaweed Jelly Recipe

This Seaweed Jelly recipe is specifically for the Herbal or Spa treatments. This translucent brown gel is made from soaked kelp seaweed, and pureed to the consistency of a Jelly. The additional liquid needed in the recipe, may be teas, distilled essences, or whatever liquid you desire. When used for Herbal treatments, it is capable of holding twice its weight in herbal essences, perfect as a poultice for problem-skin conditions. Be sure to puree the Jelly until it is very fine, so that it will wash down the drain if you choose to use it in the shower, for full body treatments.

- Dried brown Kelp Seaweed (use any amount)
- Scented Water (enough to just cover the seaweed)

Follow the Serum recipe, and soak the seaweed for at least three to five days, for it purees better when it is soft. Put the soaked seaweed pieces and liquid into a blender. Puree into a thick smooth gel. Make the jelly as thick as possible for you can always re-blend it to be thinner when you decide what treatment to do. The more you make the easier it is to blend, but even making just a small amount really only requires that you be good at pocking a spatula into the blender. Blend very well. Test by rubbing some between your fingertips. It should feel smooth with absolutely no particles.

Tips: It may be frozen for later use, or heated, for specific skin treatments and body wraps.

MAKING THE SCENTED PASTE RECIPE

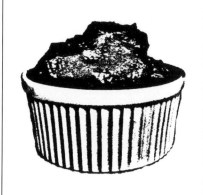

"Sensations which pertain to the Body are derived from Love and Wisdom."

- Swedenborg. 2528

3. Scented Seaweed Paste Recipe

This Seaweed Paste recipe is specifically for the Spa, and Herbal treatments. Essentially this is just soaked red or green seaweed pureed into a smooth gel. The red and green seaweeds have less gelling properties but different minerals and therefore better for specific skin-problems. The difference in the preparation is that some of the more delicate dried green and red seaweeds only need from a few hours up to a day to be fully soaked, and to be soft enough to blend into a smooth consistency. Also, some species have a very strong odor and should we rinsed first, as in the option rinsing directions.

- Dried Green or Red Seaweed
- Distilled (or Scented) Water (enough to cover the seaweed)

Follow the Serum recipe, and soak until reconstituted, from a few hours, to up to three days refrigerated. Put the softened seaweed in a blender and puree into a thick paste. Add more of the soaking liquid if needed to blend, but the thicker the better. Be sure to blend it really well.

Optional Rinsing:

Rinse the dried green and red seaweed quickly in *warm* water. Because we do not need to worry about the gelling properties with these seaweeds, the warm water helps it to soften quicker.

DISTILLATION PROCESS	
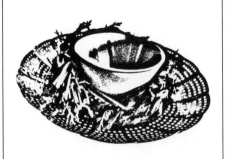	*"To Distill signifies influx and instruction, which disposes, regulates, tempers, and moderates all things."* - *Swedenborg. A.E. 594,*

This distillation process makes a clear liquid that is perfect for invisible skin-care treatments. Be sure to have plenty of ice cubes. You could also add fresh or dried flowers to mix with other herbs, and used to soak the dried seaweed, thereby creating a distilled scented Serum.

Recipe Ingredients:

- 1 bunch fresh Flowers, Herbs, or other Plants.
- 1 cup (250 ml) Water

   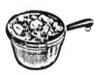

How to make:

Place a bowl on the center of a stainless steel steamer that has had its legs removed. Lay the Herbs around the edges of the bowl. Place the steamer so that it rests right on the bottom of the saucepan.

Add 1 cup (250 ml) of water and bring to a boil. Reduce to a simmer and place the lid upside down on the saucepan. Fill the lid with ice cubes (you might have to remove the lid's handle) and continue to simmer, checking every five minutes, and removing the distilled liquid, which condenses and drips into the bowl. Cool. Use this liquid to soak the dried seaweed for the Serum Recipe. Keep refrigerated.

Tips:

Do not waste the herbs or extra cooking liquid; blend the herbs for the spa treatments, or use the left-over cooking liquid for herbal treatments.

CHAPTER TWO: FACE & BODY SCRUBS

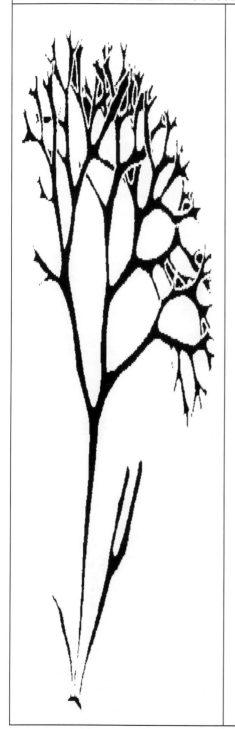

*"By
washing
the
head and hands
is understood
to purify
the internal man,
and by
washing the feet
is understood
to purify
the external."
– Swedenborg. D.P. 151*

ABOUT THE FACE & BODY SCRUBS

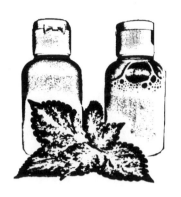

"The face corresponds to Affection."

- Swedenborg. A.E. 280

Seaweed Face & Body Scrubs

The following seaweed face and body scrubs are not any different from what you might be used to - except for the results - which are not like anything you have ever experienced. These light scrubs leave your skin feeling smooth, moisturized, and kissable.

Essentially seaweed without any other added ingredients delays the aging process because of the penetration of nutrients, anti-oxidants, minerals, and trace elements. The amino acids firm and renew tissues; the fatty acids increase fluidity to cellular membranes and help fight inflammation, while the beta-carotene slows the skin's aging, treats acne and irritated skin. Then when you add the second ingredient, which is dry, such as the salt, clay, or oatmeal, to the seaweed *Serum*, it creates an opposite combination, which would be impossible to imitate with any other ingredient. The dry ingredient removes and draws out the impurities while the seaweed replenishes the pH-balance. In the case of the oatmeal scrub, when you combine the oatmeal, especially the oatmeal milk as used here, with the seaweed Serum, the two ingredients, which are both full of good nutrients, offers a facial treatment that is pure pleasure. I hope you enjoy them!

About the Face & Body Scrubs

I have only included recipes that I have found to be perfect for mixing with seaweed jelly on my skin. I have tried other ingredients, such as bicarbonate of soda (baking soda) with seaweed S*erum* as a scrub, which totally scratched and burned my face – therefore I have not included it. You know your skin best, so feel free to change these recipes - they are only meant to be <u>examples</u> of how to use seaweed for skin-care products.

SALT SCRUB

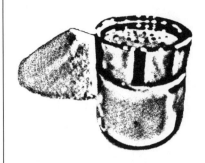

"Salt signifies the desire of conjunction of truth with good, hence nothing but salt will conjoin water, which corresponds to truth, and oil, which corresponds to good."

Swedenborg .10.300

If you have ever used a salt scrub for removing dead surface skin and dirt you know how sensitive it can be, especially on the face, one wrong move and the skin could easily be scratched – not with this salt scrub. The seaweed serum acts like a lubricating protective bubble around each salt crystal, which protects the skin while the salt conjoins to the oil to draw it deeply from the pores, leaving your skin soft and glowing – a natural circulatory stimulant. It is particularly effective for targeting problem skin areas such as the nose, where you might want to add additional salt for a second, and third scrubbing.

Recipe Ingredients:

- ¼ teaspoon (2.5 ml) Seaweed Serum
- ⅛ teaspoon (1.25 ml) Sea Salt

How to make:

Pour the seaweed jelly into the palm of one hand and sprinkle with the sea salt. Rub your hands together briefly before the salt dissolves and rub it over your entire face. Apply to either wet or dry skin.

Variations:

This salt scrub is safe for the face and around the eyes because it contains no essential oils or perfumes. If you want to add a drop or two of essential oil, feel free, but I would not recommend them be used on your face.

This salt scrub also makes an excellent full-body scrub, but for longer treatments, you might want to use a cloth or sponge brush instead of your hands.

Tips:

Keep an extra saltshaker in the bathroom for a quick face scrub.

CLAY SCRUB

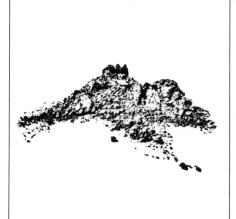

"Clay signifies the lowest natural good."

- Swedenborg. A.C. 1300

You are going to love this one for drawing oils and impurities from the skin. You can walk around the house and squint your face, the clay does not even fall off – a no-mess clay scrub, – and it's incredible.

Clay can usually be very drying to the skin, and in this recipe I used green clay which is the most drying, but with the seaweed serum, the combination leaves your skin smooth, clean, and moisturized. I have used equal parts serum and clay in this recipe, which is used immediately as a quick thinly-applied facial scrub, rubbing vigorously over the entire face. Applying more clay or more serum until the desired consistency is achieved - the thinner the mixture the better the scrub. Rinse thoroughly.

Recipe Ingredients:

- ½ teaspoon (5 ml) Seaweed Serum
- ½ teaspoon (5 ml) Green Clay Powder

How to make:

In the palm of your hand, mix a very thin consistency of the seaweed serum and the clay. Stir with your fingertips until smooth. Immediately apply a thin coat to your face with a circular rubbing motion. Rinse off with fresh water.

Variations:

This Clay scrub makes an excellent full-body scrub, but for longer treatments, you might want to use a cloth or brush instead of your hands. Also, for a clay facial masque recipe see the spa chapter.

Tips:

Keep a saltshaker filled with clay powder in the bathroom for a quick clay scrub.

OATMEAL SCRUB

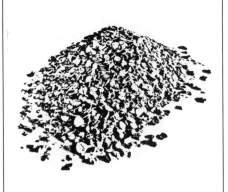

"Wheat signifies celestial love and barley spiritual love – a granary signifies heaven"

- Swedenborg 3941.

For cosmetic purposes, oatmeal is to exfoliate, to remove dead surface cells and dirt, as well as an emollient, to soothe and soften the skin. When you combine oatmeal with Kelp Serum, the mixture becomes a nutritious mineral-rich moisturizer – qualities that are difficult to obtain with any other ingredients.

This oatmeal scrub also makes an excellent less-messy invisible moisturizing treatment. Just use the oatmeal mixed with a little hot water, strain and use the oatmeal liquid to mix with the Kelp Serum for a 'heavenly' face and body moisturizing treatment.

Recipe Ingredients:

- ¼ teaspoon (2.5 ml) Seaweed Serum
- ¼ teaspoon (2.5 ml) Oatmeal (ground or strained liquid)

How to make:

Put the ground oatmeal in the center of the palm of one hand. Add the kelp jelly and rub your hands together mixing into a smooth lotion. Gently massage on your face. Allow to dry. Rinse thoroughly with fresh warm water.

Variations:

To make the invisible moisturizing mask, just make a tea using ¼ teaspoon (2.5 ml) oatmeal with 1 tablespoon (15 ml) or more boiling water. When cool, strain off a small amount of the milky oatmeal liquid to mix with ¼ teaspoon (2.5 ml) kelp jelly in the palm of your hands. Apply to your face or body, and leave on your skin as long as you like.

Tips:

You can add any of the cereal grains, even bran to this facial treatment.

MILK & HONEY PEELING SCRUB

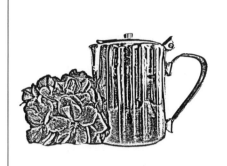

"Milk denotes the abundance of celestial spiritual things, and honey denotes the abundance of happiness and the delights thence derived"

– Swedenborg 5619

Milk and honey for cosmetic purposes is used as an emollient, to soothe and soften the skin. Essentially these ingredients correspond to purity and delight; milk to purity for it nurturing properties, and honey to delight because of it sweetness. The milk keeps the mixture moist, and the honey keeps it pliable, while the seaweed serum holds it all together.

This gentle moisturizing scrub is perfect for improving skin texture, leaving skin clear, vital and healthy. The skin becomes pH-balanced and nourished, leaving it bright and buoyant.

Recipe Ingredients:

- ¼ teaspoon (2.5 ml) Seaweed Serum
- ¼ teaspoon (2.5 ml) Milk or Cream
- ⅛ teaspoon (1.25 ml) Honey

How to make:

Mix the three ingredients in the palm of your hand into a thick lotion, and apply to your face. As it is drying, use your fingertips to rub back and forth until it rolls up and is all rubbed off. Make sure you do this over the sink. Rinse with fresh water.

Variations:

To make an invisible moisturizing mask, just eliminate the honey, and mix the milk and serum in the palm of your hands. Apply to your face or body. With this treatment, without the honey, you can leave it on your skin as long as you like.

Tips:

Any dairy product such as yogurt, sour cream, or cream cheese can be used, as well as non-dairy products such as nut, rice, or soy milk.

EXFOLIATING BODY SCRUB

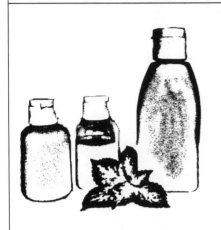

"Green, or flourishing, signifies what is alive."

- Swedenborg. A.R. 401

Green tea for cosmetic purposes is a cleanser and provides the skin with antioxidants, while the clay exfoliates, removes toxins, and improves circulation, and the seaweed supplies the minerals and nutrients to protect your skin all day long.

Use this body wash recipe either in the shower and washed off, or as a skin treatment, and allowed to dry, before washing off. This body wash is for all skin types, especially damaged and sensitive skin.

Recipe Ingredients:

- ¼ teaspoon (2.5 ml) Seaweed Serum
- ¼ teaspoon (2.5 ml) strong Green Tea
- ⅛ teaspoon (1.25 ml) Green Clay

How to make:

Mix the three ingredients in the palm of your hand and apply to your face. Alternatively, mix enough to apply to the entire body, scrubbing in a circular motion, and rinsing with fresh water.

Variations:

To make an invisible antioxidant treatment, just eliminate the clay and make a distilled green tea essence, as in the herbal treatment section. Apply to your face or body, and leave on your skin as long as you like.

Tips:

Any herbal tea will work in this recipe, just be caution that caffeine can be absorbed through the skin if you use Caffeinated tea. Alternatively, try a 'pot' treatment using marijuana stems and leaves, great for lying around all day (Ha, Ha) - but I bet it would work!

CHAPTER THREE: SKIN CARE

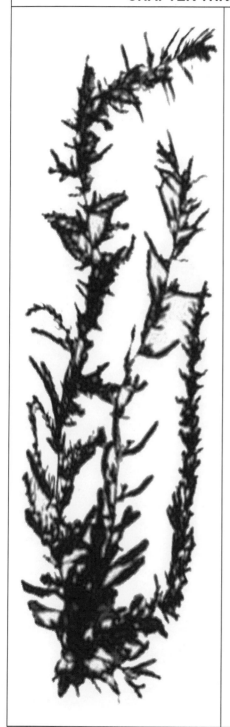

*"There are
spirits
who belong to
the province of
the skin,
especially the
rough and scaly part,
who are
disposed to reason
on all subjects,
having no perception
of what is
Good and true."*

- Swedenborg. Arcana.1835

ABOUT THE SKIN CARE RECIPES

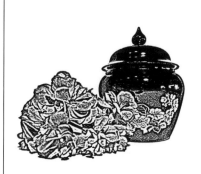

"The Skin corresponds to truth or to the false in the ultimate."

- Swedenborg. 10.036

Skin Care Jelly

Regarding the two previous quotes on the subject of 'skin', says, that if your skin is rough and scaly it represents that there is no good or truth, which is correct, since good represents oil, and truth represents water or moisture. The real meaning is that, if you 'BS' people, your skin will be rough and scaly.

Perhaps that is why there are two categories when it comes to commercial face creams – moisturizers, which correspond to 'good', and cleansers, which correspond to 'truth'. Moisturizers are gentler because of the oil or wax needed to make a creamy consistency. Cleansers, also known as toners, are clear and usually contain alcohol or other astringents that clean the pores, which allow in more moisture.

These moisturizing recipes use the seaweed *Serum*, which eliminates the need for heavy oils or wax, yet still makes a creamy consistency. These cleanser recipes use vinegar instead of alcohol, but you could also use witch hazel, which does contain a small amount of alcohol.

About the Skin Care Jelly

The base ingredient in all of these skin care recipes is the thick clear egg-white type seaweed *Serum*. Essentially, you could use just the seaweed *Serum* or *Jelly* on your skin without any of the other ingredients, for a natural organic skin treatment.

MOISTURIZING JELLY

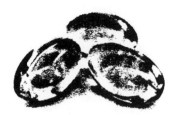

"Oil signifies the holy principle of good, or the good of love."

- Swedenborg. 3728

Vitamin E oil is usually too heavy, and too 'good' to use on the face other than for treating scars or doing intensive repair work. However, the seaweed Serum enables you to thin the Vitamin E oil to an infinitesimally small amount. Now, who would want to use any other oil but vitamin E on your face? It is incredible in small doses of 'good'. You have to try just a little.

This moisturizing jelly acts as an exfoliating and clarifying moisturizer that gently blocks impurities while vitalizing and making the skin smooth and polished. It combines the seaweed serum with Vitamin E; perfect for damaged skin and adding extra hydration, giving you a nourishing moisturizer, which encourages new cell growth. It is good for sun-damaged skin.

Recipe Ingredients:

- ½ teaspoon (2.5 ml) Distilled Rose Scented Seaweed Serum
- One-drop of edible Vitamin E Oil

How to make:

Use the smallest needle possible to poke a pinhole in the vitamin E capsule. Put the seaweed *Serum* in the palm on one hand, and squeeze one drop of vitamin E oil onto the *Serum*. Rub palms together to create a creamy lotion. Apply to face and body.

Variations:

For a more intensive private oil treatment, try using castor, halibut, or cod liver oil, instead of Vitamin E. The halibut oil is incredible, even if you can only stand the smell for an hour. When combined with the seaweed serum, it is the softest skin you will ever have.

Tips:

The fish-oil facial treatment is worth trying, if only once.

MOISTURIZING BODY SOAP

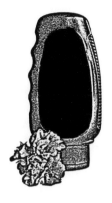

"To wash the hands and feet signify to purify the natural man, and to wash the flesh, signifies to purify the spiritual man."

- Swedenborg. A.E. 475

You might not think this is a very big deal adding green tea to soap in the mixture. However, to purify the spiritual as the quote suggests, especially after the purification of the natural man has already taken place, via the hands, has special significance. For here, we are uniting two principles, 'heat' and 'light', which correspond to love and intelligence. The green represents the light through the process of photosynthesis, as well as the 'garden', while the soap represent heat or love (good), because it is from oil, which is good.

This Moisturizing body soap is soothing and formulated with nutrient rich seaweed and natural green tea to supplement the skin's moisture balance, revitalize stressed skin, and further promote soft, youthful skin. It is suitable for all skin types. When you use this lotion, know that this mixture corresponds to 'love and intelligence united' - and corresponds to 'paradise'.

Recipe Ingredients:

- 1 Part Seaweed Serum (scented if desired)
- Five parts Castile Soap
- Ten parts Green Tea

How to make:

Make a strong green tea and mix all the ingredients in a bottle. Shake. Use in the shower. Apply to face and body.

Variations: To make an invisible antioxidant treatment, just eliminate the soap and make a scented serum, or a green tea essence, to mix with the Serum, as in the herbal treatment section. Apply to your face or body, and leave on your skin as long as you like.

Tips: Any tea will work in this recipe. Try chamomile, raspberry - even licorice.

ASTRINGENT JELLY

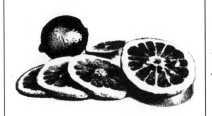

"Fruit is what the Lord gives to the celestial man, but seed producing fruit is what he gives to the spiritual man."

"Seed signifies faith grounded in charity"

- Swedenborg. 3038.

Interpreting the above quote: It restores the seed of 'faith' to your skin (truth), which prompts the cells to gratitude (to give of themselves), which becomes the fertile ground for further improvement (regeneration).

This astringent jelly uses the Serum, made from brown seaweed known to contain proven natural healing properties, and when combined with G-S-E grapefruit 'seed' extract (extract of citrus) it acts as a natural astringent to refine and tighten pores. This gentle cleanser effortlessly washes away excesses, impurities, and helps to balance the skin, clearing blemishes, and reducing skin irritations - and all without alcohol.

Recipe Ingredients:

- ½ teaspoon (2.5 ml) unscented Seaweed Serum
- 1 drop G-S-E Grapefruit Seed Extract

How to make:

Put the seaweed serum in the palm on one hand and add one drop of G-S-E Grapefruit Seed Extract. Rub the palms together to create a creamy lotion. Apply to face and body. Rinse, or leave on all day for a healing acne treatment.

Variations:

This astringent jelly is a great cleanser, scalp treatment, or anti-fungal foot lotion. It is gentle to cuts, scrapes, and all skin disorders. Apply to your face or body, and leave on your skin as long as you like. This is an instant band-aid.

Tips: The unscented Serum is best for acne or problem skin treatments, as it will cause less irritation.

SPLASH TONER RINSE

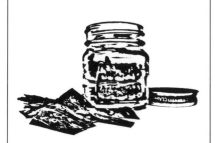

"Liquid denotes good vanishing before the heat of lust."

– Swedenborg. 8487

This splash toner uses apple-cider vinegar for its preservative and astringent properties. The lavender flower tea adds the additional liquid to make this thin enough to splash on in the shower. Healing, calming, antiseptic, nourishing, hydrating and rejuvenating are some of the words you would use to describe this super splash toner.

Used all over the body to stimulate cellular renewal and improved tightness where needed, this liquid helps to also relax muscles and joints. The nutrient rich seaweed promotes proper skin pH-balance. Apply the splash toner to your face or body, and leave on your skin as long as you like. Use it every day. It is excellent for sensitive skin.

Recipe Ingredients:

- One part Seaweed Serum
- Ten parts Lavender Flower Tea
- One part Apple-Cider Vinegar

How to make:

Make a strong lavender flower tea, and mix one part seaweed *Serum* to 10 parts tea. Add the apple-cider vinegar, and shake well. It keeps well at room temperature.

Variations:

This is a splash toner, rinsed off in the shower, leaving the skin smooth and luxuriant, with only a slight fragrance. You could also use the lavender tea to soak the seaweed, thereby starting with a scented seaweed Serum, and then add the apple-cider vinegar, which will then apply as a thick Serum.

Tips:

This recipe uses dried organic lavender flowers, but you could use any flowers. Any nice smelling herbal tea will hide the apple-cider vinegar smell.

LOTUS- ROOT UNDER-EYE SALVE

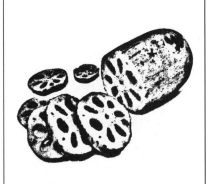

"Root signifies charity."
- Swedenborg. – A.C. 1861

This under-eye, lotus-root jelly is a soothing, fragrant free moisturizing lotion, formulated with nutrient rich seaweed, and natural lotus root to balance and revitalize sensitive skin areas and further promote soft, youthful appearance. It is suitable for all skin types, especially sensitive and grateful (charity) skin.

Recipe Ingredients:

- ½ teaspoon (2.5 ml) unscented Seaweed Serum
- ½ teaspoon (2.5 ml) steamed Lotus Root Liquid
- 10 drops Grapefruit Seed Extract- G-S-E (extract of citrus)

How to make:

Slice the unpeeled Lotus Root and place it in the bottom of a saucepan with just enough water (½ cup, 125 ml) to partially cover. Simmer until cooked. Save the liquid and pour it into a container to cool overnight. Add ten drops of G-S-E to the liquid. Shake well. Strain through a fine strainer, saving the captured white foam to apply to under the eye. Leave on as long as you like.

Variations:

Use the left-over liquid to add to any of the other treatments. Alternatively, puree the cooked root in a blender and add it to spa treatments. Apply to your face or body, and leave on your skin as long as you like.

Tips:

Using parsley as well as carrot tops created a similar white foam, but the lotus root has the best silky feeling.

MASSAGE OIL

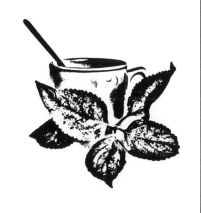

"The oil which was called the oil of holiness, was produced from olive, and mixed with aromatics."

- Swedenborg A.R. 493

Although this Massage Oil recipe is similar to the other oil based moisturizers, it deserves a page on its own. If you know of someone who does massage, you have to get them to try this combination – customers will keep coming back for more!

This is gentle, non-greasy moisturizing massage oil, formulated with nutrient rich seaweed Serum, and natural olive oil to give the ultimate massage. It maintains its moisture longer than just oil on its own, and results in a rich massage experience. Massaging this oil into the skin revitalizes, and leaves the skin softer than any oil on its own can do. It is suitable for all skin types.

Recipe Ingredients:

- One part Seaweed Serum
- Olive Oil (any amount)
- Choice of Scent

How to make:

Mix one part seaweed Serum with any amount of olive oil. You can use from as little as one-drop of oil, and thereby add more moisture from a spray bottle of water during the massage, with no oily after-effect; or add up to equal parts *Serum* and oil, thereby creating a far superior regular massage oil.

Variations:

For oily skin, or acne problem skin, just add Grapefruit seed extract with some additional moisture to keep the massage oil fluid and creamy. Apply to your face or body, massage, and leave on your skin as long as you like.

Tips:

You can use any oil with this *Serum* to make the creamiest consistency for massage oil. This massage oil recipe guarantees no more sticky skin.

ELBOWS & KNEES INTENSIVE MOISTURIZER

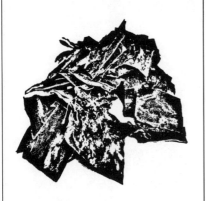

Soaked Kelp pieces

"Knees signify the conjunction of natural good with spiritual good. Bending the knee signifies acknowledgment, thanksgiving, and adoration."

– Swedenborg. - A.E. 455

This intensive moisturizer is included here because it is another way of making a Serum that is a bit thicker than the other Serum recipe. This process forms a thicker serum, applied by rubbing the wet seaweed pieces directly on your skin, under your eyes or on your elbows and knees. On its own, it does not show a vast improvement to the appearance of the skin, but it does create a smooth, soft, baby-skin 'feeling', difficult to obtain on the elbows and knees any other way.

Recipe Ingredients:

- Small pieces of Dried Kelp Seaweed
- Fresh water to Moisten

How to make:

Set aside a couple of small pieces of dried kelp. Lightly spray them on both sides with water. Put them on a plate and cover them with clear wrap. Soak for 1-5 days at room temperature. Keep them whetted down as they expand, but have no extra water on the plate. When the Serum is thick, make yourself a cup of tea, and place the plate over top of the cup to heat up the seaweed pieces. Apply hot to face and body.

Variations:

These little hot seaweed pillows make a good pore-cleaning mask if you can fix them in one spot, and allow the time for them to dry fully, without removing them to have a peek.

Tips:

You can always re-wet your face with water if you want to add a moisturizer to your elbows and knees on top of the Serum application.

CHAPTER FOUR: SUN CARE

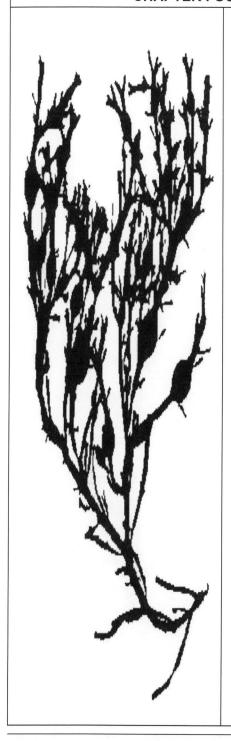

*"There are
two Suns
by which all things
were created –
the Sun
of the spiritual world
and the Sun
of the natural world;
the sun
of the natural world
was created
to act as a medium
or substitute."*

- Swedenborg
D.W.L. 153

ABOUT THE SUN CARE JELLY

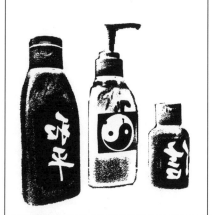

"Every man is by birth merely corporeal, and yet from corporeal he may become natural more and more interiorly, and thus rational, and at length spiritual."

– Swedenborg. C.S.L. 59

Sun Skin Care Recipes

The above is an interesting quote when you think of the Sun as signifying Regeneration, yet its heat strengthens our 'animal' nature within us, drawing it out, and through test and trial tempers it to become more rational.

This rational self eventually comprehends the natural sun as being spiritual, and the growth that its heat created, although painful, was necessary for the process that leads to this spiritual awareness.

Nothing is worse than being at the beach and sweating because of your commercial sun tan lotion. All of the seaweed sun-care recipes feel completely natural. They will not cause any sweating, and depending on how much oil you add to them, can give you a sand-free day at the beach as well, for as soon as they are dry nothing sticks to them. You will forget you have them on - this is how all sun-care products should feel - corporeal.

About the Sun Skin Care Recipes

None of these sun-care recipes contains any sunscreen or sun block, yet the seaweed seems to have a natural sunscreen, as I never burn when I wear them.

If you prefer a sunscreen, feel free to add your own, or just mix some of the Serum into your favorite sun-tan lotion, thereby you get the incredible moisturizing polished look that the Serum gives, while you stay protected.

SUNTAN LOTION

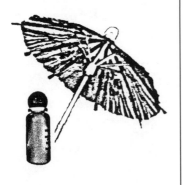

"Heat of the Sun signifies concupiscence (strong desire, esp. sexual desire, and lust) to evil, which are contained in self-love and the delights thereof."

– Swedenborg. A.R. 692

I always thought it was all the half-naked bodies during the summer that made me amorous, I never realized it was my self-love that determined my amorous response to the heat of the sun. In this recipe then, adding Coconut oil (good, love) can only magnify the natural earthy delights of sun tanning. Therefore, adding flower scent, which represents the goods of faith, helps balance the sensual influence of the oil with the faithful influence of the flowers, thereby contributing to an enjoyable stress-free day at the beach.

This Sun-tanning Serum makes your skin look and feel younger; you will forget you have it on. It re-vitalizes and deeply moisturizes even the driest skin, without any oily appearance or feeling. One application is sufficient to protect your skin for the whole day. Feel free to add your own sunscreen.

Recipe Ingredients:

- Three parts Seaweed Serum (or scented)
- One part Coconut Oil
- Choice of Scent

How to make:

Put the seaweed Serum, flower scent, and the Coconut oil in the palm of one hand. Rub hands together to create a creamy lotion. Apply to face and body. Alternatively, make up a bottle full, it will keep refrigerated for a month.

Variations:

I prefer the smell of coconut oil, but if I am going to wear this sun Serum other than at the beach then I use different oils. Try sunflower, peanut, or olive oil.

Tips: Olive oil and seaweed Serum together make the best suntan oil – try it!

SUNBURN LOTION

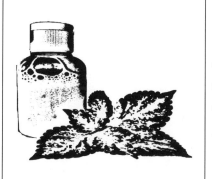

"Burning signifies damnation and punishment of evils arising from earthly and corporeal loves."

– Swedenborg. Ap. Ex. 1173

According to the above quote, sunburn is punishment from earthly pleasures, which is exactly what sunburn is, unless it is from working in the garden, but then the only way to protect from burning, would be if you <u>pretended</u> you were not really enjoying the gardening.

This Serum apple-cider vinegar combination calms, cools, and relaxes, tight, sun-burnt skin, while it subtly protects and soothes even open sores or blisters. It is non-sticky and has an invisible feeling, and other than the smell, you will never know you have it on. Re-apply as often as required to prevent pealing and flaky skin - gentle enough for the face, and for babies.

Recipe Ingredients:

- One part unscented Seaweed Serum
- One part Apple-Cider Vinegar

How to make:

Put the seaweed *Serum* and the apple-cider vinegar in the palm on one hand. Rub palms together to create a creamy lotion. Apply to face and body. Otherwise, make up any amount, enough to get you through a burn crisis, using equal parts serum and vinegar. The vinegar is a preservative and it keeps at room temperature for weeks.

Variations:

This sunburn *Serum* is good for all types of burns. Alternatively, you can add some herbs specifically for burns such as Calendula, Horse chestnut, or St. Johns Wort.

Tips:

Keep some individual portions frozen for burn emergencies. It also makes great oil-free Massage oils, for sprains and sore achy muscles.

AFTER-SUN LOTION

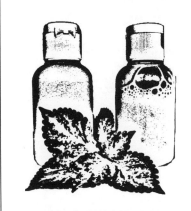

"Night signifies a state void of love and faith."

– Swedenborg. Arcana. 221

This after-sun Serum is similar to the sunburn lotion except it has no vinegar odor, and therefore better for wearing in public. It still protects your skin, while it soothes and calms the tightness due from the Sun.

The Aloe Vera is a moisturizer which firms and tones the appearance of the skin, while the seaweed serum adds nutrients and amino acids to preserve old skin cells.

Together they create a breathable moisture-protective barrier, which gives a plush clean look to the skin, with a non-greasy touch – lovable, kissable, and touchable – bring out the joy jelly!

Recipe Ingredients:

- One part scented Seaweed Serum
- One part Aloe Vera Gel

How to make:

Put the seaweed *Serum* and the Aloe Vera Gel in the palm on one hand. Rub the palms together to create a creamy lotion. Apply to face and body, again, again, and again.

Variations:

This after-sun lotion is good for all skin types. Alternatively, you can add some herbs specifically for burns such as Calendula, Horse chestnut, or St. John's Wort.

SELF-TANNING LOTION

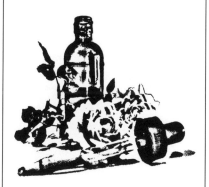

"The light of heaven effectively appears as darkness to those who are in the love of self and of the world."

– Swedenborg. Arcana 2441

This Self-Tanning Lotion was discovered completely by accident. As I was distilling some watercress, I removed the distilled clear liquid, but the remaining liquid at the bottom of the saucepan reduced to nothing, and then burnt to a mocha brown color on the bottom of the saucepan. When cooled, I mixed it with some water and some seaweed Serum, and the perfect self-tanning lotion came to be.

This Self-tanning lotion is without any chemicals, non-sticky, with a completely natural feeling. Depending on how long you let it burn in the saucepan can create even richer darker colors. When I first tried it, I applied several coats all over my face and body. That night before I got into the shower intending to go to bed, I looked in the mirror and thought I looked so good that maybe I would go out to a club. However, it was not until after I got out of the shower when I realized I had been wearing the bronzer lotion all day – and now I was pale again, so I might as well stay home.

Recipe Ingredients:

- ½ teaspoon (2.5 ml) Seaweed Jelly
- Several drops of burned liquid from a bunch of steamed Watercress

How to make:

Put a bunch of Watercress in the bottom of a saucepan, with about one half cup (125 ml) of water. Cover and simmer slowly until cooked. Remove the watercress (to use for dinner) leaving the remaining liquid. Continue to simmer uncovered, reducing the liquid, until evaporated. When completely cool, drop some water onto the burnt remnants and mix well. Refrigerate. Mix with Serum and apply.

Variations:

This self-tanning Serum makes a great face bronzer for a winter day.

Tips: Keeps refrigerated for about a month, or frozen forever.

JOY JELLY

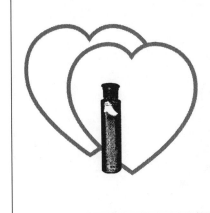

"Joy is spoken of the delight of the love of good of the heart, and of the will."

- Swedenborg A.R. 493

I have included this recipe here because it must be mentioned. Although this Joy Jell is just seaweed Serum without any other ingredient, it is not like anything that you have ever experienced before. If you are still having sex now-a-days then this lubricating jelly will make you appreciate intimacy even more. If you are not, then this joy-jelly could very well bring back an interest in sex.

This is a gentle, completely non-greasy joy-jelly, or lubricating jelly, using just the nutrient rich seaweed Serum to give the ultimate sensual experience. It is completely natural, and dries without any traces what-so-ever. It revitalizes the skin and leaves it softer than any chemically enhanced lubricating jelly. It is suitable for all sensual skin types. Just bring to room temperature and go, go, go.

Recipe Ingredients:

- One part Seaweed Serum
- Choice of Scent

How to make:

Mix one part seaweed Serum with any scent. You can add more moisture using water if it begins to dry.

Variations:

Try some mint jelly, honey, or any other of your favorite syrups, but plain is best.

Tips:

Keep some individual portions frozen in plastic wrap. They thaw immediately when dropped into hot water.

CHAPTER FIVE: BATH & SHOWER

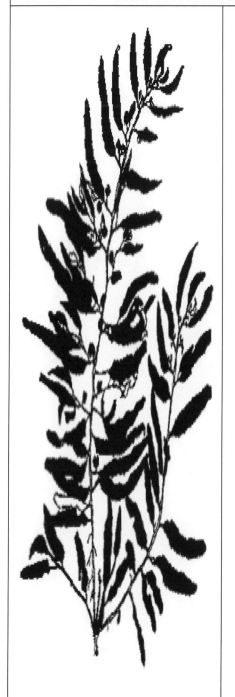

"The odor of spheres of charity and faith are perceived in another life like those of flowers, lilies, and spices."

- Swedenborg. 1519

ABOUT THE BATH & SHOWER RECIPES

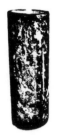
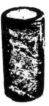

"Water signifies the spiritual things of faith. To give water signifies the common influx of truth."

– Swedenborg. 5668

Bath Care Recipes

These *bath-care* recipes are simple ways to include seaweed in your every day skin-care routine. When I began experimenting with seaweed I started to add a small amount of the serum to my store-bought skin care products for added moisturizing properties -and the effects were outstanding. Over time, the amount of Serum kept increasing until I realized that there was a limit to the amount of moisturizing effects that could be obtained by merely adding it to soap.

Although soap is the perfect preservative, and the recipes keep at room temperature for months, it is exactly that, a preservative. Therefore, if you are going to wait for the perfect store-bought seaweed *Serum* to come on the market, it will not happen without chemicals. Better to have a friend make it for you, or stick with these bath-care recipes preserved with soap.

About the Bath Care Recipes

I cannot explain why these recipes work so well, such as the deodorant, or the hair rinse. The brown kelp makes everything feel clean and moisturized.

A scientist might be able to explain why Kelp has such luxuriant qualities, but no scientist has ever been able to make broccoli last a month at room temperature without adding many chemicals. Seaweed is just the same as broccoli, best when it is fresh or dried and second best, when it is frozen – preserved any other way will need chemicals.

Therefore these recipes are the recommended proportions to add to your bath products, and for more dramatic moisturizing effects you will have to move on to the other chapters, which include more skin-friendly ingredients.

NATURAL BATH SACHETS

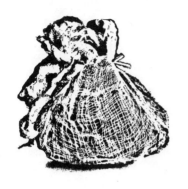

"A bath signifies truth from good."

– Swedenborg. Ap.Ex. 675

The ultimate tool in Thalassic (seaweed, seawater) therapy, contains seaweed blended with sea salt. The marine minerals and chlorophyll assist the organic cells to fight off microbes and boost the body's metabolism, improves circulation, and rejuvenates the skin's surface. This bath treatment is ideal for all skin types including those with skin disorders.

Recipe Ingredients:

- Spent soaked Seaweed
- 2 cups (500 ml) Sea Salt
- Fragrance of Choice

How to make:

This bath treatment uses the leftover seaweed from the serum recipe. Lay a piece of tin foil onto the counter-top, and add cheesecloth on top of it. Use several layers of cheesecloth, as it is weak and tears easily when wet.

Dump the spent soaked seaweed leftovers on top of the cheesecloth. Add the sea salt and any other ingredients. Wrap and tie the cheesecloth, and bundle it in the tin foil. Freeze until set. When ready to use, take it out of the freezer and remove the tin foil. Place the tied seaweed-filled cheesecloth into the bath under the hot water as it is filling. Enjoy!

Variations:

You can add any ingredients such as Epson salts, bicarbonate of soda, fresh and dried flowers or herbs to the cheesecloth sachet.

Tips:

Use cheesecloth instead of muslin, because the larger holes in the cheesecloth allow the seaweed jells to more easily release in the bath.

HAND & BODY SOAP

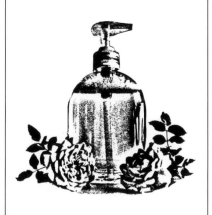

"Soap denotes the good by which purification is effected."

– Swedenborg. A.E. 475

Although the hands get good 'taking-care-of' throughout this skin-care regime, this Liquid Hand and Body Soap Serum is so simple to use yet thoroughly moisturizes as it cleans - a daily hand-care regime without any bother, without any refrigeration.

The soap to Serum ratio in this recipe is ideal for dry and chapped hands. I prefer to use Castile soaps for the body, but for the hands, any liquid hand soap will work. The soap acts as a preservative, and will keep at room temperature for a month without spoiling.

Recipe Ingredients:

- One part Seaweed Serum
- Ten parts Castile Soap

How to make:

Just add the seaweed Serum to the Castile soap, or store bought liquid hand soap and shake or mix well.

Variations:

If you are using the Castile soap, it works great as a shower wash. It also makes a good shaving lotion, not very foamy, but a soft, soft, soft shave. Apply to your face or body, and rinse thoroughly.

Tips:

If you desire, use a scented Castile soap, or add the seaweed Serum to your hair shampoo. It is safe enough to add to baby shampoo.

BABY POWDER DEODORANT JELLY

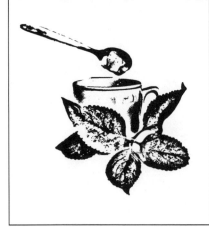

"To be cleansed signifies to be sanctified."

– Swedenborg.- A.C. 4545

When I wear antiperspirant, my feet start to sweat within three days. Even deodorants can be non-effective despite their peculiar scents. So imagine the delight to find a deodorant that works.

This Baby-Powder Jelly is a great under-arm deodorant, it is non-sticky, completely unnoticeable, and you can only smell it up very close. It is a delicate, every day deodorant that keeps you smelling nice all day, and leaves your skin fresh and dry. All skin types, excellent for sensitive skin. This is a far better way to put baby powder on a baby as well - with no dust flying around.

Recipe Ingredients:

- One part Seaweed Serum
- One part Baby Powder

How to make:

Put the seaweed Serum in a cup, and sprinkle the baby powder on top. Stir with a spoon until thick and creamy. Put some jelly on the back of the spoon, and apply it to the underarms using the back of the spoon.

Variations:

For a more moisture-absorbing deodorant, try adding a little white clay.

Tips:

This baby-powder deodorant keeps for a couple of days, but turns brown after the third day, even refrigerated. Therefore, it needs to be prepared fresh.

MOISTURIZING HAIR RINSE

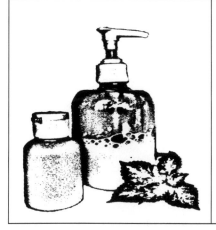

"The head of a man signifies the all of his life which has relation to love and wisdom."

– Swedenborg. - A.R. 476

This is a moisturizing hair rinse made from brown seaweed, which contains proven anti-septic, anti-inflammatory, anti-bacterial, and natural healing properties.

The seaweed contributes the rich moisturizing properties to this formula, and when blended with the apple-cider vinegar, a natural astringent, it rinses away excess oil and impurities, and helps balance the skin. It also clears blemishes and reduces skin irritations, without the use of alcohol.

Recipe Ingredients:

- One part Seaweed Serum
- One part Apple-Cider Vinegar
- 10 parts Rosemary or Nettle Tea
- Choice of Scent

How to make:

Mix the seaweed Serum, apple-cider vinegar and tea in a bottle and shake. The apple-cider vinegar acts as a preservative, therefore it can be at room temperature without spoiling. Keep it by the shower for a quick hair rinse.

Variations:

You can substitute the apple-cider vinegar for any other vinegar. In addition, you could eliminate the vinegar, using just the tea, which will give you a more moisture-absorbing body rinse.

Tips:

This hair rinse keeps for a month.

TOOTH-PASTE POLISH

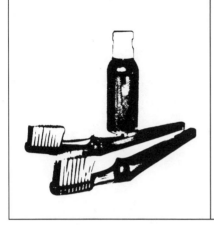

"Teeth signify the ultimate of the life of the natural man, which is called sensual - the lowest natural principle."

– Swedenborg. - A.E. 435

This delicate, every day tooth polish contains seaweed and bicarbonate of soda to lightly clean tooth surface without any harsh scrubbing effects. Excellent for sensitive teeth, it will leave your teeth refreshed and healthy.

This is not my favorite recipe as the seaweed serum is not very pleasant tasting, but when you compare it to regular toothpaste, you realize how much flavoring regular toothpaste has in it, and any alternative would be better than the chemicals used in regular toothpaste.

Recipe Ingredients:

- One part scented Seaweed Serum
- One part Bicarbonate of Soda
- Peppermint

How to make:

Use either a distilled peppermint essence, or a peppermint tea, to soak the seaweed to make the scented Serum. Put the scented seaweed Serum, and the bicarbonate of soda in a cup and mix thoroughly.

Variations:

For a more stain removing toothpaste, add some sea salt.

Tips:

This toothpaste keeps for a couple of days, therefore, it needs to be prepared fresh.

CHAPTER SIX: SPA TREATMENTS

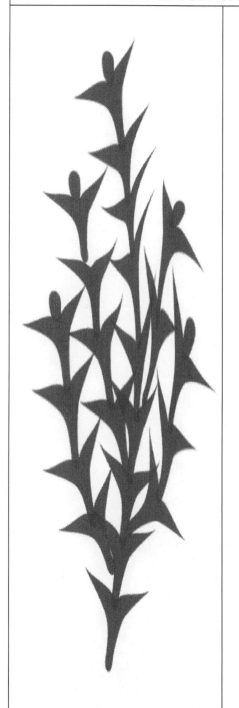

"The body is an organ composed of all the most mysterious things which are in the world of nature."

(Swedenborg A.C. 4523)

HEALING SPA TREATMENTS

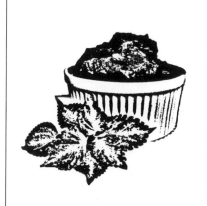

"Minerals are the substances which compose the forms of the animal and vegetable kingdoms."

– *Swedenborg. - A.Cr. 96*

Algotherapy : Seaweed Spa Treatments

Algotherapy is a luxuriant skin treatment therapy. It uses seaweed in the bath, or applied to the skin as a warm paste and then wrapped, even applied as a herbal poultice, which is absorbed through the skin. The *Paste* has a longer drying time than the *Jelly*, therefore, depending on what other ingredients you mix with it, such as clay, oil, or herbs, can result in deep pore cleaning, or very deep moisturizing treatments – excellent for problem-skin therapy used with the herbal treatments.

The recipes in this chapter use unprocessed seaweed Paste made from pureed seaweed - not seaweed extracts. These treatments are very intense. Think of them as $1,000 an ounce, better than any commercial chemically treated spa product, unless they make their own like this.

Adding Red & Green Seaweeds to your Spa Treatments

The Brown Seaweeds offer-up luxuriant sensual gelling and moisturizing gels, whereas the red and green seaweeds contain additional minerals and nutrients, more preferable for medicinal treatments. Therefore, mixing the different species together means we obtain the luxuriant sensual texture of the brown kelp, but improve the medicinal properties by adding another species, either red or green.

These Spa treatments are the area to add any of the many other varieties of seaweed to your mix. Since the Spa treatments are applied warm the results can be quite spectacular, in fact elbows and knees respond really well to this type of deep moisturizing treatment. Try it - you will be amazed!

REFORMATION FACIAL MASK

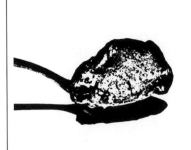

*"... and made **clay** of the spittle, and anointed the eyes of the blind man with the clay, by which was signified reformation by truths from the letter of the Word."*

– Swedenborg.- A.E. 239

This Reformation Clay Facial Mask corresponds to the 'lowest natural good' we can experience on the physical plane before it is considered a 'sin'. Now I understand why clay can be so corrosive, and how that corrosive property draws out the last bit of dirt – thereby setting us free to sin again.

In the above quote, clay reforms by representing the 'letter of the word', which initiates the reformation, the first act of a new birth. Clay then is our last resort - which points us anew – a 'kind of healing'. Since 'sin' is "returning in memory to a previous pleasurable experience which disturbs our peace of mind," clay helps us leave behind those memories of debauch, so that we can sin and love again. Enjoy!

Recipe Ingredients:

- 1 part brown Seaweed Jelly
- 4 parts green Seaweed Paste
- 1 part green Clay

How to make:

Put the seaweed Serum, Paste and clay in a jar and stir until smooth. Set the jar in a sink of hot water. Apply to face as a warm thick paste, with a little scrubbing. Allow to completely dry, before removing with water.

Variations:

This mask is not messy once you have it on. In fact, when it dries, it stays moist working to build new skin. This is another seaweed pampering session with no mess.

Tips:

You will need straws for your cocktails with this mask - and not too much laughing, we do not want to wrinkle the mask. Waiter... a straw please!

MOISTURIZING DETOX BATH

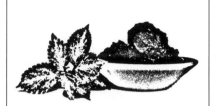

"To draw water signifies to be instructed"
– *Swedenborg. 3057.*

It has been a long day, sixteen hours, fed up, exhausted, and a sore back. I took a Seaweed bath, and now I am writing about it, fully refreshed. Incredible, it drew out all those complaints.

The green seaweed takes this to a new level of therapy. The Kelp makes it luxurious, and added with the green seaweed, makes it a highly therapeutic blend to detoxify and stimulate circulation. Used hot in the bath creates a full body treatment for swollen areas, cellulite, skin disorders, and dehydration or just for an extra boost of essential nutrients to the skin. This bath soak leaves epidermis incredibly soft, smooth, firm, fresh, and rejuvenated. Use once a week to ensure moisture levels of the skin are balanced, and to relieve those achy-back days – it did mine! Soak until instructed.

Recipe Ingredients:

- 1 part Brown Seaweed Jelly
- 4 parts Green Seaweed Paste
- 1 part Lavender Tea

How to make:

Mix the seaweed Jelly, Paste, and lavender tea together, until smooth. Pour mixture into a hot bath, and mix until dissolved.

Variations:

This is a fabulous way to have this kind of deep seaweed therapy with no mess. It washes right down the drain. Imagine your own spa treatment in the comfort of your home – this is it! Try adding a little bubble bath and you will not notice the green specks floating around. This is the softest my skin has felt since experimenting with all of these recipes.

Tips: You do not need any oil added to this bath treatment, just candles and cocktails - waiter! It would make a great 'mud-wrestling' jelly too!

FACE & BODY POLISH

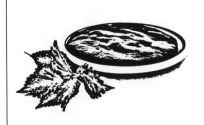

"Heavenly peace flows in, when the lusts arising from the love of self and of the world are taken away."

– Swedenborg. 5662

Shut the curtains, turn up the thermostat, and run a hot bath. Apply this polish to your entire body, and run around the house naked so you can leave it on as long as possible. Wash it off in a hot bath, and have kissable soft skin again.

This exfoliating and clarifying body polish gently removes impurities while vitalizing and making the skin smooth and polished. The two different seaweeds blend very well for extra hydration, while the sea salt and the Vitamin E oil creates a nourishing polish that loosens dead cells and encourages new cell growth.

Recipe Ingredients:

- 1 part brown Seaweed Serum or Jelly
- 4 parts green Seaweed Paste
- ½ part Sea Salt
- One Vitamin E Oil Capsule

How to make:

Put the seaweed Serum or Jelly, green seaweed Paste, sea salt, and Vitamin E oil in a container. Heat the mixture by setting the container in a sink full of hot water. Apply to face and body. Leave on as long as possible. Lie in the sun and use a spray bottle of water to re-moisten, and then let dry, then re-moisten, and dry again.

Variations:

This is a fabulous way to deep clean the pores and moisturize at the same time, and again without a lot of mess. It stays on the skin and washes down the drain. Imagine moisture rich skin again – this is it! Try other oils as well, for the sea salt helps to remove any excess oil, leaving your skin extremely silky smooth. Tips: Finish up with a scented body wash.

WRINKLE-REDUCING BODY TREATMENT

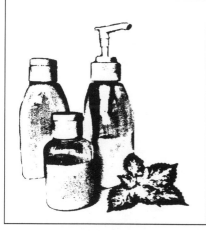

"A state of Youth corresponds to the affection of good and truth."

– Swedenborg. 3254

This is a wrinkle-reducing seaweed body-treatment to calm and nurture the skin. Apply it gently all over the body, one half hour before getting in a hot bath, or shower. The seaweed supplies the skin with antioxidants and minerals to moisturize and balance the skin's pH to promote a healthy younger looking complexion. The Grapefruit Seed Extract (G-S-E) acts as an exfoliating cleanser to assist in removing toxins. It is gentle enough to use several times a week, for all skin types, especially sun-damaged, dehydrated, or mature. For an extra boost, follow up with an application of the Seaweed Serum.

Recipe Ingredients:

- 1 part Seaweed Jelly
- 2 parts Green Seaweed Paste
- Several drops of Grapefruit Seed Extract (G-S-E)

How to make:

Put the seaweed jelly, paste, and G-S-E in a container or jar, mix well, and cover. Place the covered container in a sink full of hot water until warm. Apply warm to face and body, to wear as a pretreatment before getting in a hot bath to soak and to wash it off.

Variations:

This deep cleans and sterilizes problem skin, such as acne or eczema conditions. It moisturizes without added oil, generally not tolerated for acne problems. The G-S-E helps to remove any excess oil, leaving your skin extremely silky smooth and clean.

Tips:

For acne or other similar skin conditions, apply like a mudpack without rubbing. Finish up with a scented body wash.

NEUTRALIZING RED SEAWEED TREATMENT

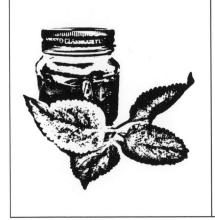

"Red is predicated of the good of love, because it proceeds from the fire of the spiritual sun."

– Swedenborg. A.R.167

This is a moisturizing, healing, and detoxifying seaweed treatment. It is dark red and applies like a thin paste. It is unlike any of the other treatments. The raw red seaweed has little or no gelling properties until boiled, but the mineral properties feel completely different on the skin. The circulation is stimulated, and the skin is softens. It has the anti-inflammatory as well as anti-microbial effects, and is a treatment to calm inflamed tissue and to prevent premature aging.

Recipe Ingredients:

- One part Seaweed Jelly
- Two parts Red Seaweed Paste
- ½ part milk, cream, or yogurt. (Optional)

How to make:

Put the brown seaweed jelly, red seaweed paste, and cream in a container or jar, mix well, and cover. Place the covered container in a sink full of hot water until warm. Apply warm to face and body, to wear as a pretreatment before getting in a hot bath to soak and then to wash it off.

Variations:

Generally, this treatment feels like a medicinal treatment, because of the smell. The red seaweed has a decidedly stronger salty odor than the other seaweeds, so be prepared. Eliminate the milk, and use this treatment for an acne treatment as well.

Tips:

This red seaweed treatment would be great mixed with stimulating spices to hide the odor. Finish up with a scented body wash.

CHAPTER SEVEN: HERBAL BEAUTY TREATMENTS

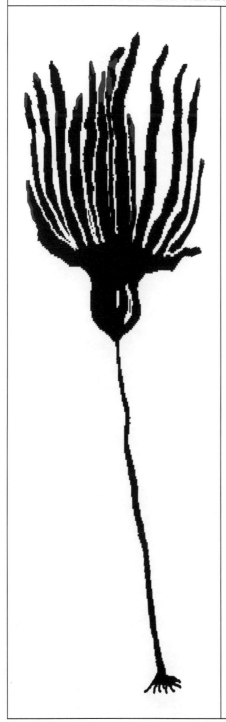

*"The number
seven
was esteemed
holy,
as is well known,
by reason of the
six days of creation,
and of the
seventh,
which is the
celestial man,
in whom is
peace, rest,
and the
Sabbath."*

- Swedenborg A.R.657.

HERBAL BEAUTY TREATMENTS

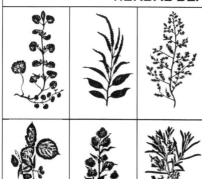

"Every herb, in the word, signifies some species of Scientifics."

- Swedenborg. A.C. 7626

Herbal Beauty Treatments: Inner Beauty

In Metaphysics, it is believed that we absorb one third of what we 'need' through the food we eat, one third through the thoughts we think, and one third through our skin. This chapter is about improving the absorption and expiration through our skin to strengthen our inner beauty first.(the next chapter is focused on outer beauty).

In this chapter, I have used seaweed Serum in a way to demonstrate its 'suspension dispersion' properties, which gives seaweed Serum the ability to disperse herbal essences uniformly within an invisible pH-balanced coating. When applied to the skin, it offers the opportunity to focus on specific issues using different herbal treatments at the same time.

All of these recipes use the distillation process (as discussed in chapter one), to make the herbal essences for these treatments. This process makes a clear liquid, safe to use on the face, even around the eyes. You may also choose to make a strong tea or hot water infusion, but teas usually obtain some color, which can stain the skin, which is OK if you are sitting around home, but might be a little 'green' for going out to a club. On the other hand, you may also choose to use herbs in their raw state, but do a skin test before applying them to your face.

About the Herbal Beauty Treatments

Use either the *Serum* or the *Jelly* for these herbal treatments. The *Serum* is for invisible all-day or all-night skin-treatments, whereas the *Jelly* is more for relaxing problem-skin bath treatments. Seaweed as a base ensures that your skin stays well moisturized and hydrated, while actively fighting the signs of aging and promoting a younger, fresher looking complexion.

| SEVEN PRINCIPLES OF CELLULAR REGENERATION |

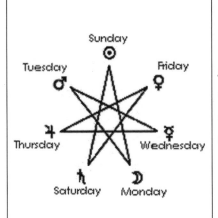

The Heptagram is a geometrical formula that represents the seven creative principles of regeneration in perfect balance.

– a symbol of perfection!

The Seven Days of the Week

Nicholas Culpepers' (1616-1654) pioneering work on classifying herbs is the foundation of herbal medicine. But he also developed another little known classification, based on each herb being governed by one of the seven personal planets.

In Alchemy, these seven planets, represent the seven inner 'metals', that when brought into balance, make the universal medicine, the Elixir of Life. Although in Alchemy, we are talking about becoming "eternal" - our skin cells regenerate in exactly the same way, from the inside out.

Each of the seven planets also rules over one of the seven days of the week. The 'seven days' of the week correspond to the work of 'regeneration', which essentially is the elimination of negativity within the personality.

This following seven Seaweed Jelly Treatments are for treating inner, 'spiritual' issues – which if not corrected, could eventually lead to dis-ease.

The ruling planet reveals the herb's 'hidden' properties. Just as herbs are harvested at specific times, assigning the herb to a specific day, it now becomes possible to determine the most propitious time for its administration.

This little-used planetary classification now makes it very easy to choose the right herb in all instances. It also makes it fun to experiment. You could use a fun Venus herb on a strife-full Monday or an intellectually stimulating Mercury Herb for an exam on Thursday, or a peaceful Moon Herb for a serious Saturday.

BEAUTY BALANCING TREATMENTS				
Week Day	Ruler	Metal	Sin	Opposite Attributes
Sunday	☉ Sun	Gold	Pride	Regeneration - Fertility & Sterility
Monday	☽ Moon	Silver	Sloth	Memory - Peace & Strife
Tuesday	♂ Mars	Iron	Wrath	Awakening - Grace & Sin
Wednesday	☿ Mercury	Quicksilver	Envy	Attention - Life & Death
Thursday	♃ Jupiter	Tin	Gluttony	Rotation - Wealth & Poverty
Friday	♀ Venus	Copper	Lust	Imagination - Wisdom & Folly
Saturday	♄ Saturn	Lead	Greed	Cosmic Consciousness - Dominion & Slavery

Seven Days of the Week: Ruling Metal

The planets, or the seven inner creative principles, are also, dual in nature. According to Paul Foster Case in his book The Tarot, they are associated with a pair of opposites, and these opposites give a clue to their spiritual meaning, and therefore the correct remedy.

Each day of the week is ruled by one of the seven 'inner' metals. Sunday which is ruled by the Sun, corresponds to the metal 'Gold', and although the Sun represents the 'heart' of the physical body, as the metal Gold, it corresponds with the 'Higher Self'. Therefore the Sun herbs have the ability to influence us on a much deeper level when used on its ruling day.

Balancing The Seven Inner Metals

Our skin is a reflection of our personality. Swedenborg says, "the skin corresponds to the truth and the false in the ultimate". This means, that if our skin is rough and dry, then to improve it, we must correct the rough and dry aspects of our personality, such as our prudishness, or our uncaring attitude. If our skin is smooth and clammy, we must deal with the smooth and clammy aspects of our personality, such as our integrity or our sponginess. Even if our skin is too oily, it could mean that we are too sticky or too co-dependent.

Therefore, when balancing the seven metals, first determine if you demonstrate the positive, or the negative qualities. If you lack pride, you would use a Sun Herb Jelly on Sunday, or every day to increase the pride in your life, or until the condition improves.

SUNDAY'S REGENERATING JELLY

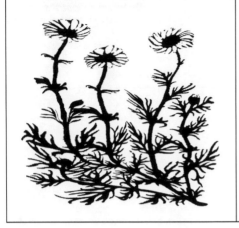

"The Sun signifies celestial and spiritual love, and in an opposite sense, self-love and its lusts."

- Swedenborg. 2441

This Sunday-Treatment uses the Sun-Herb Chamomile, but all of the Sun-herbs re-vitalize and stimulate as they subtly uplift and regenerate the skin. The Sun's essential nature is to radiate perfect beauty, strength, and confidence throughout the entire circulatory system. The Sun's spiritual energy increases generosity and love, which receives consideration and optimistic responses in return.

The Sun-herbs act to balance a lack of the spiritual energy, which causes the negative traits related to self-love, such as vanity, arrogance, over-optimism, and excessive pride by bringing about a strengthened inner core, with greater spiritual awareness, resulting in softer, smoother skin.

The opposite attributes of Fertility & Sterility in relation to the Sun-herbs is one of perspective. For as we try to improve the softness of our skin by outer means, it is not until we improve the inner-skin of our personality that we begin to understand the shift in perspective that is necessary to improve any outward condition.

This shift in perspective - the 'Gold' - is a new concept of personality that begins the process of cellular regeneration. This new self-identification is transferred onto newly developed fertile cells, which eventually liberates us from physical circumstances. The golden age was a time of innocence – the primary principle of regeneration - when we <u>knew</u> we were loved.

Recipe Ingredients:
- ½ teaspoon (2.5 ml) Seaweed Serum
- ½ teaspoon (2.5 ml) distilled essence of Chamomile
- A touch of Egg White

How to make:
Put the seaweed jelly and the Sun-Herb essence in the palm on one hand. Dip the tip of one fingertip of the other hand into some raw egg white briefly. Rub palms together to create a creamy lotion. Apply to face and body.

SUN HERBS

Regeneration – Principles of Fertility & Sterility

"Regeneration - by which the new intellectual principle and the new will principle are formed." - Swedenborg. 5354.

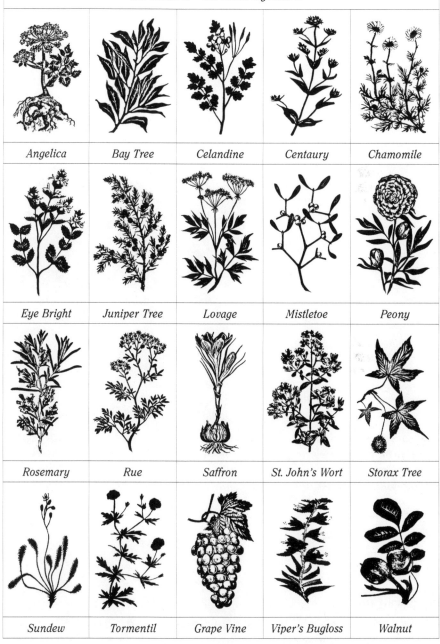

Angelica	Bay Tree	Celandine	Centaury	Chamomile
Eye Bright	Juniper Tree	Lovage	Mistletoe	Peony
Rosemary	Rue	Saffron	St. John's Wort	Storax Tree
Sundew	Tormentil	Grape Vine	Viper's Bugloss	Walnut

MONDAY'S NURTURING JELLY

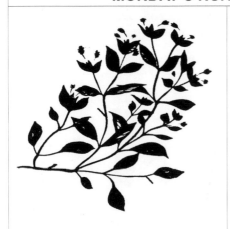

"The reason time appears to be something, is owning to the mind's reflecting on those things which are not objects of affection, or love".

- Swedenborg. 3827

This Monday-Treatment uses the Moon-Herb Chickweed, which calms and cools the feelings and emotions. All Moon-herbs bring contentment and relaxation by quieting the memory, and as the tension thoughts subside, a restful coordinating feeling is felt, restoring harmony and rhythm to the cells of the Lymphatic system.

The Moon herbs also act to balance a lack of the Moon's spiritual energy, which causes the negative traits related to idleness, sadness, apathy, or illusions. This self-sedating effect transforms the emotions into a deep empathic feeling for others - an increased sensitivity without the over emotionalism, or the fearfulness and melancholy that caring more for others can often cause.

The opposite attributes of Peace & Strife in relation to the Moon-herbs is one of calming the memory through faith. The Memory, at its deepest level of the subconscious mind, is a virgin state of peace, which corresponds to 'spiritual faith'. All of the levels above that are, in an opposite sense, also related to faith, but faith derived from man's own intelligence, otherwise felt as Strife.

The 'Silver' in relationship to the Memory represents truth. Truth or 'silver' flows through memory, and at its deepest level is true, and its upper level is false. When the 'silver' has been purified, or the 'spiritual faith' is brought to the surface, there is a union of the positive with the negative - and the faith becomes love – and all manner of creative manifesting power is restored. "Until the Moon is not" (Ps. lxii. 5)

Recipe Ingredients:

- ½ teaspoon (2.5 ml) Seaweed Serum
- ½ teaspoon (2.5 ml) distilled essence of Chickweed

How to make:

Put the seaweed jelly and the Moon-Herb essence in the palm on one hand. Rub palms together to create a creamy lotion. Apply to face and body.

MOON HERBS

Memory – Principles of Peace & Strife

"The Memory is only the entrance into man, and as a courtyard, by which there is entrance to a house." - Swedenborg. A.E 290.

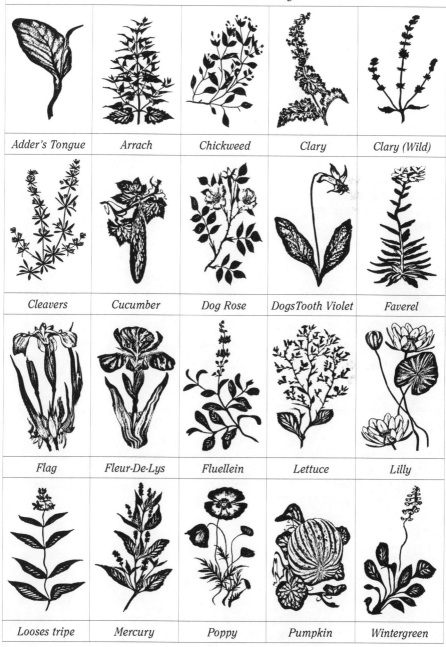

Adder's Tongue	Arrach	Chickweed	Clary	Clary (Wild)
Cleavers	Cucumber	Dog Rose	DogsTooth Violet	Faverel
Flag	Fleur-De-Lys	Fluellein	Lettuce	Lilly
Loosestripe	Mercury	Poppy	Pumpkin	Wintergreen

TUESDAY'S AWAKENING JELLY

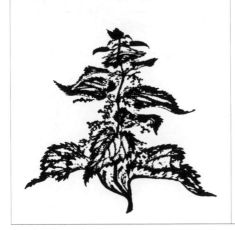

"Mars - the spirits who inhabit that planet are amongst the best of all spirits, and have relation to thought grounded in affection,"

- Swedenborg. E.U.88

This Tuesday-Treatment uses the Mars-Herb Nettle, which initiates new cell life, and improves the Muscular System. All Mars-herbs energize and intensify the need to act, to feel, to live. They activate the generative organs, which lift us out of lethargy and inertia, increasing spontaneity and drive - sluggishness be gone! Use Mars-herbs for initiating new action, or a situation that requires leadership and dominion – such as a first date, a second date, and a third date.

The Mars-herbs also act to balance a lack of the Mar's spiritual energy, which causes the negative traits of anger, hatred, cruelty, and wrath by getting the energy moving and thereby curtailing frustration.

The opposite attributes of Grace & Sin in relation to the Mars-herbs is one of right action. Action represents 'Iron', and corresponds to 'rational' truth. When the 'silver' or truth, from the previous Moon principle has not been fully purified, there is an identification with our thoughts and ideas 'as if' they are our own, and therefore us. This false identification with our ideas creates a loss of rational truth, and therefore a loss of Grace. But this misconception also separates us from others, and from our 'Gold', and more importantly forces us to hover in the realm of sensual truth, otherwise called Sin – where we believe that anyone who questions our ideas, is actually attacking us. The resulting storms and battles that ensue, built by words from a lack of rational truth eventually causes a lightning flash of awakening, freeing us from our false identification and driving us in search of our 'gold'- and more illumination – hence Mar's connection with awakening.

Recipe Ingredients:

- ½ teaspoon (2.5 ml) Seaweed Serum
- ½ teaspoon (2.5 ml) distilled essence of Stinging Nettle

How to make: Put the seaweed jelly and the Mars-herb essence in the palm on one hand. Rub palms together to create a creamy lotion. Apply to face and body.

MARS HERBS

Mars: Awakening – Principles of Grace & Sin

"To Awaken denotes a state of illustration, which flows into the natural man, when it is initiated in good." - Swedenborg. 2185

Anemone	*Arssmart*	*Barberry*	*Basil*	*Brook-Lime*
Bryony	*Butcher's Broom*	*Chives*	*Flax weed*	*Garlic*
Gentian	*Honeysuckle*	*Hops*	*Hyssop*	*Onion*
Pepper	*Radish*	*Rhubarb*	*Sarsaparilla*	*Tarragon*

WEDNESDAY'S STIMULATING JELLY

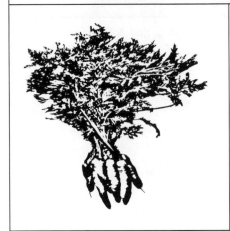

"Mercury has relation to the memory of things abstracted from what is material. Material things are in themselves fixed, stated, and measurable."

- Swedenborg. E.U.10.

This Wednesday-Treatment uses the Mercury-Herb Carrot, which improves mental alertness, reasoning, and intelligence. All Mercury-herbs stimulate optimism and contribute to emotional balance by better concentration, thus increased skill in writing and orderliness. Mercury-herbs are a cure for despondency and indecision, It tempers over-activity of negative emotions, restoring balance, and resulting in mental poise and an altruistic attitude.

The Mercury-herbs also act to balance a lack of Mercury's spiritual energy, which causes the negative traits of malice, envy, falsehood, and dishonesty, by shifting perspective, and resulting in improved clarity.

The opposite attributes of Life & Death in relationship to the Mercury-herbs is connected with focusing our attention more spiritually. When the previous phase has cleared our identification with thoughts and ideas, our attention is able to focus upon the object with such clarity that we begin to see into it its spiritual essence, and thereby bring it to Life. The mind is then a clear channel, and wherever the mind goes, healing follows – the healing being, the recognition of the objects' spiritual essence, or 'Gold'.

The Mercury metal is Quicksilver, which is a liquid at room temperature, and represents the fluidity of mind and its ability to become the object of its focus. When we can see in others their spiritual essence, it reflects the good and truth flowing through us, and prepares and opens the internal spiritual level of mind, and despite the appearance, we are able to experience the good and truth in all.

Recipe Ingredients:

- ½ teaspoon (2.5 ml) Seaweed Serum
- ½ teaspoon (2.5 ml) distilled essence of Carrot Tops

How to make: Put the seaweed jelly and the Mercury-herb essence in the palm on one hand. Rub palms together to create a creamy lotion. Apply to face and body.

MERCURY HERBS

Mercury: Attention – Principles of Life & Death

"The truly spiritual states are very easy: one is simply, here Now!"
(Elisabeth Haich - Sexual Energy and Yoga.)

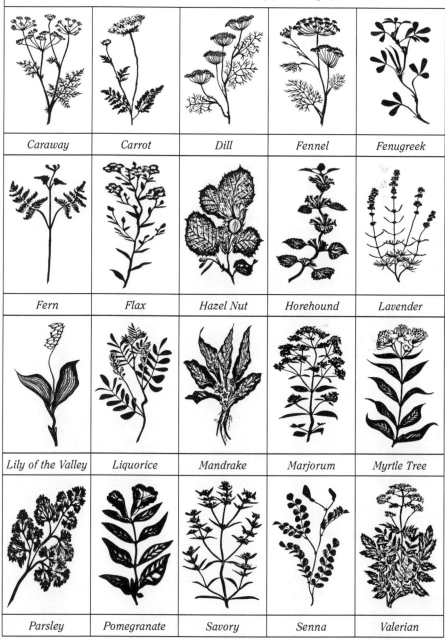

Caraway	Carrot	Dill	Fennel	Fenugreek
Fern	Flax	Hazel Nut	Horehound	Lavender
Lily of the Valley	Liquorice	Mandrake	Marjorum	Myrtle Tree
Parsley	Pomegranate	Savory	Senna	Valerian

CHAPTER SEVEN: HERBAL BEAUTY TREATMENTS - 67

THURSDAY'S REGULATING JELLY

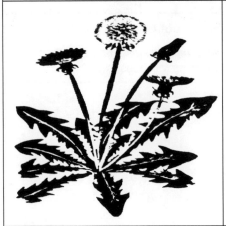

"Jupiter consists of thinking well and justly on all occasions of life. Those do not die of diseases, but in tranquility, as in sleep"

- Swedenborg. E.U. 62, 84

This Thursday-Treatment uses the Jupiter-Herb Dandelion. All Jupiter-herbs regulate the flow of fluids by a mild stimulating antiseptic manner, and relives congestion, especially in the digestive system. Jupiter-herbs have an affinity with natural order, and thus improve the appreciation for all life, thereby drawing greater goodness into itself, experienced as charity to others, greater abundance for thyself, and a beneficent aura that draws all good things to it – both material and spiritual.

The Jupiter-herbs also act to balance a lack of Jupiter's spiritual energy, which causes the negative traits of bigotry, hypocrisy, and gluttony by bringing some sort of conciliation.

The opposite attributes of Wealth & Poverty in relationship to the Jupiter-herbs is connected with cause and consequence. When the previous phase has strengthened our ability to see the spiritual essence or 'gold' in all things, and it is reflected as our ability to experience the good and truth in all, then we are struck by a deep gratitude for, and connection to, all life, including our cycles of poverty. For it is in our cycles of pain, that we learn acceptance, and with acceptance develops the beneficent aura which ends the cycle of selfishness, and we begin to love others as ourselves, which alleviates loneliness, and begins to attract to us all good things.

Tin has reference to the natural or external circumstances, and it is only when this is conjoined with the internal, the ability to see the essence, is man blessed and happy, effected only by charity, and only by the 'Gold'.

Recipe Ingredients:

- ½ teaspoon (2.5 ml) Seaweed Serum
- ½ teaspoon (2.5 ml) distilled essence of Dandelion

How to make:

Put the seaweed jelly and the Jupiter-herb essence in the palm of one hand. Rub palms together and apply to your face or body as often as needed.

JUPITER HERBS 4

Jupiter: Rotation – Principles of Wealth & Poverty

"Where love rules, there is no will to power, and where power predominates, love is lacking. The one is the shadow of the other." - Carl Jung.

Agrimony	Asparagus	Beets	Betony	Bilberries
Borage	Chervil	Chestnut Tree	Cinquefoil	Costmary
Dandelion	Dock	Endive	Fig Tree	Hyssop
Jessamine	Sage	Samphire	Swallow Wort	Thorn Apple

CHAPTER SEVEN: HERBAL BEAUTY TREATMENTS - 69

FRIDAY'S PAMPERING JELLY

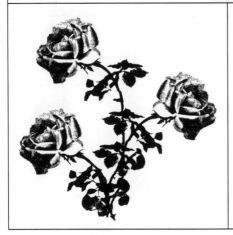

"In the planet Venus there are two kinds of men, of tempers and dispositions opposite to each other, the first, mild and humane, and second, savage and almost brutal."

- Swedenborg E.U. 105-109

This pampering Friday-Treatment uses the Venus-Herb Rose. Venus-herbs are mildly sedative and depressant, creating a relaxing effect until the nerves become quiet, and the emotions are balanced. Then the attractive force strengthens, and the imagination stimulated. This new fuller affection power, the attractive force of the universe, can now touch others by your increased capacity to love. Affection now becomes the creating principle, and emotion drives us to our goal effortlessly.

The Venus-herbs also act to balance a lack of Venus's spiritual energy, which causes the negative traits of lust, unchaste behavior, and eroticism by attracting appropriate relationships, and bringing greater pleasure.

The opposite attributes of Wisdom & Folly in relationship to the Venus-herbs is in reference to the use of our imagination. When the previous phase has strengthened our ability to see the beauty in all experiences because of our deep gratitude for all life, and we begin to attract to ourselves all good things, because we feel blessed and happy, is when our 'Copper', or imagination, is put to the test and purified.

Copper has reference to 'natural' good, which is emotionally charged personal desire, which is not good, unless it is made spiritual good, which is creative love. Natural good is our response to attracting 'all good things' and identifying the source as if from ourselves - hence folly. Spiritual good is our response to the essence or 'gold' we see in others, which stirs an emotion within us, which radiates love to serve others. In this way, we enjoy the blessedness of all good things, without attachment - hence creative love.

Recipe Ingredients:

- ½ teaspoon (2.5 ml) Seaweed Serum
- ½ teaspoon (2.5 ml) distilled essence of Rose

How to make: Put the seaweed jelly Herb essence in the palm on one hand. Rub palms together and apply to your face or body as often as needed.

| VENUS HERBS | |

Venus: Imagination – Principles of Wisdom & Folly

"Innocence is the essential principle of regeneration."
- Emanuel Swedenborg. 3994

Alder	Alehoof	Archangel	Beans (Broad)	Blackberry
Burdock	Cherries	Colt's Foot	Columbine	Daffodil
Figwort	Foxglove	Golden Rod	Kidney-wort	Mint
Primrose	Rose	Sorrel	Thyme	Vervain

SATURDAY'S STABILIZING JELLY

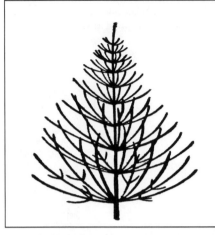

"The inhabitants of this planet are upright and modest. In acts of divine worship they are exceedingly humble, and at such times the divine beams forth from the face and affects the mind."
- Swedenborg E.U. 97.

This stabilizing Saturday-Treatment uses the Saturn-Herb-Horsetail. All Saturn-herbs stabilize, and slow down any degenerative tissue damage. They promote clean healing of wounds by confining and limiting in their slightly stimulating but antiseptic effect. They bring emotional control by inhibiting anxious, materialistic anxieties, and suspicious inhibitions.

The Saturn-herbs also act to balance a lack of Saturn's spiritual energy, which causes the negative traits of greed, treachery, and covetousness by relieving the fear, and thereby bringing greater discipline and responsibility. These herbs also operate to remove blockages to the excretory system.

The opposite attributes of Dominion & Slavery in relationship to the Saturn-herbs is in reference to our perspective of limitations. When the previous phase has strengthened our ability to love without attachment, we feel blessed and happy because the love radiates from within us, as opposed to us seeking it from without. For when someone seeks love from others, increasing our love toward them merely strengthens their slavery aspect, and then they use their love or possessions to dominate others.

The metal Lead, has reference to sensual truth. When we understand the use of limitation, it strengthens our concentration, and allows us to reach the interior center, or peace of the 'here and now', and escape the bondage that materialistic slavery creates. It is our salvation from death, death being, unable to see the essence of life. When dominion is established by the use of self-imposed limitation, it allows us to experience a state of Nirvana, the peace that enables us to start fresh on a new higher arc of the Sun cycle.

Recipe Ingredients:

- ½ teaspoon (2.5 ml) Seaweed Serum
- ½ teaspoon (2.5 ml) distilled essence of Horsetail

How to make: Put the Serum and Herb essence in the palm on one hand. Rub palms together and apply to your face or body as often as needed.

SATURN HERBS

Saturn: Cosmic Consciousness – Principles of Dominion & Slavery

"The dominion of self-love is infernal, but the love of dominion grounded in the love of uses, is heavenly." - Swedenborg. CSL 261

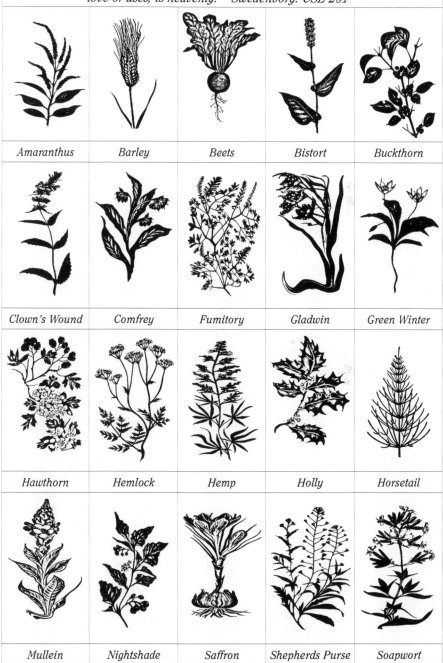

Amaranthus	Barley	Beets	Bistort	Buckthorn
Clown's Wound	Comfrey	Fumitory	Gladwin	Green Winter
Hawthorn	Hemlock	Hemp	Holly	Horsetail
Mullein	Nightshade	Saffron	Shepherds Purse	Soapwort

BEAVTY BALANCING-TREATMENTS				
Week Day	Planet	Sun Sign	Opposite Sign	Opposite Planet
Sunday	☉ Sun	Leo	Aquarius	Saturn
Monday	☽ Moon	Cancer	Capricorn	Saturn
Tuesday	♂ Mars	Aries Scorpio	Libra Taurus	Venus Venus
Wednesday	☿ Mercury	Virgo Gemini	Pisces Sagittarius	Jupiter Jupiter
Thursday	♃ Jupiter	Sagittarius	Gemini	Mercury
Friday	♀ Venus	Taurus Libra	Scorpio Aries	Mars Mars
Saturday	♄ Saturn	Capricorn	Cancer	Moon

Finding the Opposite Planet: The Herbal Remedy

I have included the above chart to help you find the opposite planet, and thereby the opposite herb to be used as the balancing herbal remedy. This opposite Remedy Treatment is still for treating the spiritual aspect, or the inner issue, to help the cells remember their true purpose - to regenerate - and maintain perfect beauty.

If you determined that you were overbalanced and demonstrated the negative Sun traits such as vanity, arrogance, or excessive pride you would strengthen the opposite metal, to correct that particular issue. By using the Sun as an example, the Sun, rules the zodiacal sign Leo, its' opposite sign is Aquarius, ruled by Saturn. Only the traditional rulers are used in this formula, Uranus co-rules, but Saturn is the traditional ruler of Aquarius.

Therefore, seaweed Serum mixed with a Saturn herb, and applied to the skin, would be used to tone-down any extremes in relation to the issues ruled by the Sun. Applied on a Sunday, would be considered a light treatment, and applied on a Saturday, Saturn's ruling day, would be the opposite and strongest treatment.

The same logic would apply to giving treatments based on the ruling hour of the day. (see chart: planetary hour ruler). Applied during a Sun hour would be a light positive treatment, and applied during a Saturn hour, a strong counter-treatment.

CHAPTER EIGHT: HOMEOPATHIC HEALING

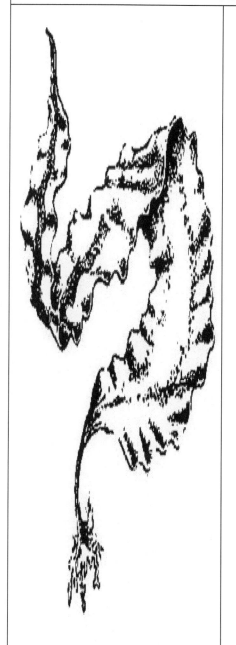

"It is only when the blood is chemically perfect that the full quota of Spirit, otherwise God-power, can enter the body, for "Like attracts like."

- The Zodiac and the Salts of Salvation: by George Washington Carey.

HOMEOPATHIC ENERGY MEDICINES

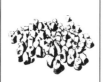

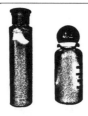
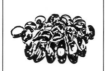

"Medicines:

evils and falses take away health from the internal man and induce sickness in the mind, the hence pains."

- Swedenborg. 6502

The Twelve Outer Skin Areas

The previous chapter dealt with the seven days, or the seven principles of regeneration. The inner metals must be balanced first, before any outer skin problems can be diagnosed accurately.

This chapter deals with the outer skin, the 'physical' body, which is divided into twelve areas, and corresponds to the twelve astrological signs, or colors, as well as the twelve homeopathic cell salts. To use these twelve possible skin treatments, first note which area of the body has the problem, then find its ruling astrological sign, or color, and then determine the opposite sign or color, to use as the balancing remedy.

Seaweed Serum: Color Therapy Medium

In this chapter, I have used seaweed Serum to demonstrate seaweeds' 'suspension vibration' properties, which gives seaweed Serum the ability to become 'like' the vibratory essence that it is exposed to.

Perhaps this theory would be easier to understand if you were to think about just adding food coloring to the seaweed Serum, which would change its' color vibration - but I do not recommend that you apply that to your skin.

Perhaps this is why seaweed extracts are so widely used in the pharmaceutical industry, for their ability to 'take on' another vibration, such as growing bacteria in a petri dish.

How I use seaweed serum as a color therapy medium is, I like to have some clear Serum sitting on my window-sill for a few hours in a Red colored bottle, until it 'becomes' a Mars Exercise Jelly that I apply all over my skin, before I go jogging. Sometimes when I apply the red 'imbued' Serum, I feel my skin actually absorbing energy. All the colors are worth trying!

SKIN AREA CORRESPONDENCES		
SIGN	COLOR	SKIN AREA
Aries	Red	*Head above brow, ear openings.*
Taurus	Red-Orange	*Neck, throat, lower jaw*
Gemini	Orange	*Hands, arms, shoulders*
Cancer	Orange-Yellow	*Chest, mammary glands*
Leo	Yellow	*Dorsal spine region*
Virgo	Yellow-Green	*Upper abdominal*
Libra	Green	*Lumbar spine region*
Scorpio	Green-Blue	*Nose, genito-urinary, rectum*
Sagittarius	Blue	*Hips, thighs*
Capricorn	Blue-Violet	*Knees, skin as organ*
Aquarius	Violet	*Ankles to knees*
Pisces	Red-Violet	*Feet, toes.*

Seaweed Serum: A Healing Medium

Seaweed Serum is also perfect for sterile environments, such as applying it on burns or other broken skin problems. I do not know of any other product or ingredient that you can put on your skin and not feel it.

I would classify Seaweed Serum as being vibration-ally sensitive, in that it can be prepared hot or cold, or used as a carrier for other energy medicines, such as sound therapy. I can imagine laying in a bath full of warm seaweed Serum (would cost a lot of money) and have some piano music vibrating through the seaweed jelly into my soul.

Finding the Opposite Sign: The Color Remedy

I have included a Skin Area Correspondence chart to determine the ruling color of each surface skin-area of the body. As an example of how to use the chart, suppose your hands were always very dry. Gemini, the color Orange, rules the hands, and we know from the Planetary Opposite Chart in the previous Herbal medicine chapter, that Gemini's opposite sign is Sagittarius, which is Blue - so you would use a Blue imbued Seaweed Serum, to correct the dry hands problem.

This color therapy technique is for healing physical diseases. Suppose you had hair-scalp problems, ruled by Aries and the color Red, whose opposite sign is Libra, the color Green. Use a Green imbued seaweed Serum or Paste for perhaps a hair rinse, or a spa scalp treatment.

HOMEOPATHIC CELL-SALT TONIC JELLY

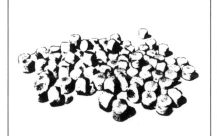

"Minerals are the substances which compose the forms of the animal and vegetable kingdoms."

- Swedenborg. - A. Cr. 96

This homeopathic cell-salt tonic jelly is included here because it is a fragrant free alternative therapeutic lotion, formulated to supply mineral compounds (or mineral salts) to various parts of the body via the skin. The seaweed Serum permits the solution to linger on the skin waiting for absorption and assimilation of the salt into the cells of the body.

You will need to know more about homeopathic cell salts for an expanded use of this treatment, but for this example I have used the Bio- plasma (12 in 1) balanced combination which includes all 12 tissue salts as a general skin tonic, guaranteed to restore any mineral deficiency. It is suitable for restoring balance to all skin types.

Recipe Ingredients:
- ½ teaspoon (2.5 ml) Seaweed Serum
- 4-6 Bio-plasma (12 in 1) Homeopathic Cell Salt Tablets

How to make:

Put the seaweed *Serum* and the Homeopathic Cell Salt tablets in the palm of one hand. Rub palms together to create a creamy lotion. Apply to face and body.

TWELVE HOMEOPATHIC CELL SALTS	
Kali Phosphoricum -*Potassium Phosphate*	Natrum Phosphoricum -*Sodium Phosphate*
Natrum Sulphuricum - *Sodium Sulphate*	Calcarea Sulphurica -*Calcium Sulphate*
Kali Muriaticum -*Potassium Chloride*	Silicea -*Silica, Oxide of Silicon*
Calcarea Fluorica -*Calcium Fluoride*	Calcarea Phosphorica -*Calcium Phosphate*
Magnesia Phosphorica -*Magnesium Phosphate*	Natrum Muriaticum -*Sodium Chloride,*
Kali Sulphuricum -*Potassium Sulphate*	Ferrum Phosphoricum -*Iron Phosphate*

CELL SALT : CORRESPONDENCE		
Cell Salt	*Sun Sign*	*Planet*
Kali Phosphoricum -Potassium Phosphate	Aries	**Mars**
Natrum Sulphuricum - Sodium Sulphate	Taurus	**Venus**
Kali Muriaticum -Potassium Chloride	Gemini	**Mercury**
Calcarea Fluorica -Calcium Fluoride	Cancer	**Moon**
Magnesia Phosphorica -Magnesium Phosphate	Leo	**Sun**
Kali Sulphuricum -Potassium Sulphate	Virgo	**Mercury**
Natrum Phosphoricum -Sodium Phosphate	Libra	**Venus**
Calcarea Sulphurica -Calcium Sulphate	Scorpio	**Mars**
Silicea -Silica, Oxide of Silicon	Sagittarius	**Jupiter**
Calcarea Phosphorica -Calcium Phosphate	Capricorn	**Saturn**
Natrum Muriaticum -Sodium Chloride,	Aquarius	**Saturn**
Ferrum Phosphoricum -Iron Phosphate	Pisces	**Jupiter**

Cell Salts Correspondence: Healing Technique

I have included a Homeopathic Cell Salts Correspondence Chart in case you find using Cell Salts an easier method than herbs, for resolving particular complicated skin problems.

Sometimes determining whether a skin problem is because of a food reaction, or merely a reaction to some laundry detergent, or shower soap, can be a difficult task. By applying the mineral deficiency, or its opposite, as a skin application mixed with the seaweed serum, can help avoid the confusion.

One way I test cell salts is, if they appear to have a taste, then my body needs them. If they taste bland, then my body does not need that mineral. I have kept the Bio 12 combination cell salts on-hand, and taken them internally off and on for over thirty-five years. I find, as an example, when nothing else seems to relieve a sore back, homeopathic cell salts do help.

Summation

Like I said previously, one way I tested these seaweed recipes was to try them on my own skin. And the only reason I have included the additional healing modalities such as the herbal medicine, or the color therapy, is in the hope that it might encourage you to try these seaweed formulas on your own skin problem.

Enjoy!

Source: *Cell salt, sun sign correspondences from: The Zodiac and the salts of Salvation - Homeopathic Remedies for the Sign Types - George Washington Carey & Inez Eudora Perry, First published 1932 by Samuel Weiser, Inc.*

BIBLIOGRAPHY

Algae to the rescue! : everything you need to know about nutritional blue-green algae	Abrams, Karl J
Anita Guyton's anti-wrinkle plan : how to have smoother, more youthful skin in just 30 days.	Guyton, Anita.
An Introduction to Macrobiotics: A Beginners Guide to the Natural Way of Health	Heidenry, Carolyn.
Apple Cider Vinegar: Health System,/	Bragg, Paul & Patricia.
Back to Eden	Kloss, Jethro.
Brown algae : structure, ultrastructure and reproduction	Vijayaraghavan, M. R.
Complete book of beauty treatments : everything you need to know about the latest products and methods	Sedgbeer, Sandra.
Creating your own cosmetics-- naturally : the alternative to today's harmful cosmetic products	Smeh, Nikolaus J.
Culpeper's color herbal	Culpeper, Nicholas, 1616-1654.
Culpeper's complete herbal	Culpeper, Nicholas, 1616-1654.
Culpeper's medicine : a practice of Western holistic medicine	Tobyn, Graeme.
Down-to-earth beauty : a lavish guide to natural cosmetics, scents, potpourris, love charms, and potions	/by Palmer, Catherine.
Easy beauty recipes : making your own personal-care products in minutes for pennies	Jager, Mariah, 1969-
Esoteric Keys of Alchemy,	Case, Paul Foster
The encyclopedia of healing plants : a guide to aromatherapy, flower essences & herbal remedies	Wildwood, Christine.
The green beauty Bible : the ultimate guide to being naturally gorgeous	Stacey, Sarah.
The green beauty guide : your essential resource to organic and natural skin care, hair care, makeup, and fragrances.	Gabriel, Julie
Handmade medicines : simple recipes for herbal health /by Hobbs, Christopher, 1944-	Hobbs, Christopher, 1944-
Health and beauty the natural way	Purchon, Nerys.
The herbal home spa : naturally refreshing wraps, rubs, lotions, masks, oils, and scrubs Greta.	Breedlove,
Herbs : growing & using the plants of romance	Varney, Bill.

BIBLIOGRAPHY

Herbs, their culture and uses	by Clarkson, Rosetta E
How to Heal with Color	Andrews, Ted
How to make your own herbal cosmetics : the natural way to beauty	Sanderson, Liz.
Inspirational Thoughts On The Tarot	Rev. Ann Davies
Lotions, oils and essences : bathroom and beauty products from natural ingredients /	Rippin, Joanne.
Lotions, oils and essences : bathroom and beauty products from natural ingredients /	Rippin, Joanne.
Medical botany : plants affecting human health	Lewis, Walter Hepworth.
The mixer, hand mixer, and blender cookbook	Culinary Arts Institute.
Modern & healthy body care : recipes for professional, natural skin and hair care products	Bombeli, Karin.
The natural beauty & bath book : nature's luxurious recipes for body & skin care	Kellar, Casey.
Natural beauty : making and using simple beauty products	Duff, Gail.
Natural beauty : pamper yourself with salon secrets at home.	DuPriest, Laura
Natural beauty basics : create your own cosmetics and body care products	Byers, Dorie.
Natural beauty for all seasons : more than 250 simple recipes and gift-giving ideas for year-round beauty	Cox, Janice.
Natural beauty from the garden : more than 200 do-it-yourself beauty recipes and garden ideas	Cox, Janice
Natural beauty recipe book : how to make your own organic cosmetics and beauty products	Farrer-Halls, Gill.
Organic at home /by Hill, Diana.	
Pacific seaweeds: a guide to common seaweeds of the West Coast	by Druehl, Louis D., 1936-
Perfect Balance: Ayurvedic Nutrition For Mind, Body, and Soul,	Atreya
Production and utilization of products from commercial seaweeds.	McHugh, Dennis J.
Properties and products of algae; proceedings.	Symposium Culture of Algae
Rosemary Gladstar's herbal recipes for vibrant health : 175 teas, tonics, oils, salves, tinctures, and other natural remedies for the entire family.	Gladstar, Rosemary.

BIBLIOGRAPHY

Rosemary Gladstar's herbs for natural beauty.	Gladstar, Rosemary.
Rosemary Gladstar's herbs for natural beauty.	Gladstar, Rosemary.
Sea vegetable celebration : [discover seaweed's healing benefits and easy use in over 100 vegetarian recipes]	Erhart, Shep.
Sea vegetables : harvesting guide & cookbook.	McConnaughey, Evelyn
Seafood sense : the truth about seafood nutrition & safety	Babal, Ken.
Seaweed : nature's secret to balancing your metabolism, fighting disease, and revitalizing body & mind	Cooksley, Valerie Gennari.
Seaweeds and their uses	Chapman, V.J. 1910-
Seaweeds : a color-coded, illustrated guide to common marine plants of the east coast of the United States	Hillson, Charles James, 1926
Self Healing Yoga & Destiny	Haich, Elisabeth & Yesudian, Selvarajan.
Sexual Energy and Yoga,	Haich, Elisabeth
Single-celled organisms.	Pascoe, Elaine
Tarot and individuation : a Jungian study of correspondences with cabala, alchemy, and the chakras	Gad, Irene, 1925-
Thai spa book : the natural Asian way to health and beauty	Jotisalikorn, Chami.
Through the gates of death	Fortune, Dion.
The Complete Book of Energy Medicines: Choosing your path to health,	Dziemido, Helen E., M.D.
The Message of the Stars,	Heindel, Max & Augusta
The Mystical Quabalah	Fortune, Dion
The Tao of Medicine: Ginseng and Other Chinese Herbs for Inner Equilibrium and Immune Power	Fulder, Stephen, Ph.D.
The Tarot,	Case, Paul Foster

BIBLIOGRAPHY

The training & work of an initiate.	Fortune, Dion.
The ultimate natural beauty book : 100 gorgeous beauty products to make easily at home	Fairley, Josephine.
The Zodiac and the Salts of Salvation : Homeopathic Remedies for the Sign Types,	Carey, George Washington & Perry, Inez Eudora
Yoga : uniting East and West /	Yesudian, Selva Raja.
Inspirational Thoughts On The Tarot	Rev. Ann Davies

SUN HERBS LATIN NAMES

Angelica – *Angelica Archangelica*	Rosemary – *Rosmarinus Officinalis*
Bay Tree – *Laurus Nobilis*	Rue (Garden) – *Ruta Graveolens*
Celandine (The Greater) *Chelidonium Majus*	Saffron – *Crocus Sativus*
Centaury – *Centaurium Erythraea*	St. John's Wort – *Hypericum Perforatum*
Chamomile – *Chanaemelum Nobile*	Storax Tree – *Styrax Officinalis*
EyeBright – *Euphrasia Officinalis*	Sundew – *Drosera Anglica*
Juniper Tree – *Juniperus Communis*	Tormentil – *Potentilla Erecta*
Lovage – *Levisticum Officinale*	Vine Tree – *Vitis Vinifera*
Mistletoe – *Viscum Album*	Viper's Bugloss – *Echium Vulgare*
Paeony – *Paeonia Officinalis*	Walnut – *Juglans Regia*

MOON HERBS LATIN NAMES

Adder's Tongue – *Ophioglossum Vulgatum*	Flag (Yellow) – *Iris pseudacorus*
Arrach (Garden) – *Atriplex Hortensis*	Fleur-De-Lys (Garden/ Blue) *Iris Germanica*
Chickweed – *Stellaria Media*	Fluellein, Paul's Betony, *Veronica Officin*
Clary – *Salvia Sclarea*	Lettuce (Common Garden) – *Lactuca Sativa*
Clary (Wild) – *Salvia Verbenaca*	Lily (Water Garden) – *Lilium Candidum*
Cleavers – *Galium Aparine*	Loosestrife – *Lysimachia Vulgaris*
Cucumber – *Cucumis Sativus*	Mercury (French) – *Mercurialis Annua*
Dog Rose – *Rosa Canina*	Poppy (Wild) – *Papaver Phoeas*
Dog's Tooth Violet – *Erythronium Densanis*	Pumpkin – *Cucurbita Pepo*
Faverel (Wooly) – *Draba Incana*	Wintergreen – *Pyrola Minor*

MARS HERBS LATIN NAMES

Anemone – *Anemone Nemorosa*	Gentian (Autumn) – *Gentianella Amarella*
Arssmart (Hot & Mild) – *Polygonum*	Honeysuckle – *Lonicera Periclymenum*
Barberry – *Berberis Vulgaris*	Hops – *Humulus Lupulus*
Basil – *Ocymum Basilicum*	Hyssop (Hedge) – *Gratiola Officinalis*
Brook-Lime – *Veronica Beccabunga*	Onion – *Allium Cepa*
Bryony – *Bryonia Dioica*	Pepper – *Piper Nigrum*
Butcher's Broom – *Ruscus Aculeatus*	Radish (Garden) - *Raphanus Sativus*
Chives – *Allium Schoenoprasum*	Rhubarb – *Rheum Rhaponticum*
Flaxweed – *Linaria Vulgaris*	Sarsparilla – *Smilax*
Garlic – *Allium Saticam*	Tarragon - *Artemisia Dracunculus*

MERCURY HERBS LATIN NAMES

Caraway – *Carum Carvi*	Lily Of The Valley – *Convallaria Majalis*
Carrot (Wild) – *Daucus Carota*	Liquorice – *Glycyrrhiza Glabra*
Dill – *Anethium Graveolens*	Mandrake – *Mandragora Officinarum*
Fennel – *Foeniculum Vulgare*	Marjoram (Common) – *Organum Vulgare*
Fenugreek – *Trigonella Foenum-Graecum*	Myrtle Tree – *Myrtus Communis*
Fern (Brake Bracken) *Pteridium Aquilinum*	Parsley (Common) – *Petroselinum Crispum*
Flax – *Linum Usitatissimum*	Pomegranate Tree – *Punica Granatum*
Hazel Nut – *Corylus Avellana*	Senna (Red flowered) – *Colutea Orientalis*
Horehound (Black) - *Ballota Nigra*	Savory (Summer) – *Satureia Hortensis*
Lavender – *Santolina Chanaecyparissus*	Valerian (True Wild) – *Valeriana Officinalis*

JUPITER HERBS LATIN NAMES	
Agrimony - *Agrimonia Eupatoria*	Dandelion – *Taraxacum Officinale*
Asparagus – *Officinalis & Sativus*	Dock (Common) – *Rumex Obtusifolius*
Beets (White) – *Beta*	Endive – *Cichorium Endivia*
Betony (Water) – *Betonica Aquatica*	Fig Tree – *Ficus Carica*
Bilberries – *Vaccinium Myrtillus*	Hyssop – *Hyssopus Officinalis*
Borage – *Borago Officinalis*	Jessamine – *Jasminum Officinale*
Chervil – *Myrrhis Odorata*	Sage (Common Garden) – *Salvia Officinalis*
Chestnut Tree – *Castanea Sativa*	Samphire - *Crithum Maritimum*
Cinquefoil – *Potentilla reptans*	Swallow-Wort – *Asclepias Syriaca*
Costmary – *Balsamita Major*	Thorn-Apple – *Datura Stramonium*
VENUS HERBS LATIN NAMES	
Alder (Common) – *Alnus Glutinosa*	Figwort – *Scrophularia Nodosa*
Alehoof – *Glechoma Hederacea*	Foxglove – *Digitalis Purpurea*
Archangel – *Lamium*	Golden Rod – *Solidago Virgaurea*
Beans (Broad) – *Vicia Faba*	Kidneywort – *Umbilicus Rupestris*
Blackberry – *Rubus Fructicosus*	Mint Garden, Pepper, Spear- *Mentha Spicata*
Burdock (Greater) – *Arctium Lappa*	Primrose – *Primula Vulgaris*
Cherries (Winter) – *Physalis Alkekengi*	Rose (Damask) – *Rosa Damascena*
Colt's Foot – *Tussilago Farfara*	Sorrel (Common) – *Rumex Acetosa*
Columbine – *Aquilegia Vulgaris*	Thyme (Wild) – *Thymus Serpyllum*
Daffodil – *Marcissus Pseudonarcissus*	Vervain (Common) – *Verbena Officinalis*
SATURN HERBS LATIN NAMES	
Amaranthus – *Amaranthis Hybridus*	Hawthorn – *Hieracium Murorum*
Barley - *Hordeum Vulgare*	Hemlock – *Conium Maculatum*
Beets (Red) – *Beta*	Hemp – *Cannabis Sativa*
Bistort – *Polygonum Bistorta*	Holly – *Ilex Aquifolium*
Buckthorn – *Rhamnus Catharticus*	Horsetail – *Equisetum Arvense*
Clown's Woundwort – *Stachys Palustris*	Mullein (Black) – *Verbascum Nigrum*
Comfrey – *Symphytum Officinale*	Nightshade (Common) – *Solanum Nigrum*
Fumitory – *Fumaria Officinalis*	Saffron (Meadow) – *Colchicum Autumnale*
Gladwin – *Iris Foetidisima*	Shepherd'd Purse *Capsella Bursa-Pastoris*
Green (Winter) – *Trientalis Europaea*	Soapwort – *Saponaria Officinalis*

Source: Culpeper's complete herbal - Culpeper, Nicholas, 1616-1654.

PLANETARY HOURS

HOURS' RULING PLANET

Hour	Sunday	Monday	Tuesday	Wednesday	Thursday	Friday	Saturday
1	☉	☽	♂	☿	♃	♀	♄
2	♀	♄	☉	☽	♂	☿	♃
3	☿	♃	♀	♄	☉	☽	♂
4	☽	♂	☿	♃	♀	♄	☉
5	♄	☉	☽	♂	☿	♃	♀
6	♃	♀	♄	☉	☽	♂	☿
7	♂	☿	♃	♀	♄	☉	☽
8	☉	☽	♂	☿	♃	♀	♄
9	♀	♄	☉	☽	♂	☿	♃
10	☿	♃	♀	♄	☉	☽	♂
11	☽	♂	☿	♃	♀	♄	☉
12	♄	☉	☽	♂	☿	♃	♀
13	♃	♀	♄	☉	☽	♂	☿
14	♂	☿	♃	♀	♄	☉	☽
15	☉	☽	♂	☿	♃	♀	♄
16	♀	♄	☉	☽	♂	☿	♃
17	☿	♃	♀	♄	☉	☽	♂
18	☽	♂	☿	♃	♀	♄	☉
19	♄	☉	☽	♂	☿	♃	♀
20	♃	♀	♄	☉	☽	♂	☿
21	♂	☿	♃	♀	♄	☉	☽
22	☉	☽	♂	☿	♃	♀	♄
23	♀	♄	☉	☽	♂	☿	♃
24	☿	♃	♀	♄	☉	☽	♂

Source: Planetary Hours - re-written from Wikipedia

NUTRITIONAL CHART: COMPARISON		
COMPONENT	KELP	CABBAGE
Protein	3.03	1.21
Lipid	0.64	0.18
Digestible Carbohydrate	0	5.37
Fibre	9.68	0.8
Iodine	0.21	0
Calcium	0.15	0.47
Iron	0	0.01
Magnesium	0.11	0.02
Phosphorus	0.08	0.02
Sodium	0.87	0.02
Potassium	0.05	0.25
Zinc	0	0
Manganese	0	0
Ascorbic Acid	0	0.05
Alpha-Tocoperol	0	0
Thiamin	0	0
Riboflavin	0	0
Niacin	0	0
Folic Acid	0.05	0.25
Cholesterol	0	0
Leucine	0.26	0.06
Lysine	0.11	0.06
Phenylalanine	0.11	0.04
Glycine	0.11	0.03
Alanine	0.14	0.04
Valine	0.21	0.05

APPROXIMATE CONCENTRATIONS OF SOME COMPONENTS OF KELP AND, FOR COMPARISON, CABBAGE (values are % of dry weight).
Reference: Composition of Foods. Agriculture Handbook No. 8-11 U.S. Department of Agriculture, Human Nutrition Information Service 502 pp. (1984)

NUTRITIONAL CHART: SEAWEED, KELP, RAW

Nutrient	Units	Value per 100 grams	# of Data Points	Std. Error
Approximates				
Water	g	81.58	8	1.75
Energy	kcal	43	0	0
Energy	kj	180	0	0
Protein	g	1.68	3	0.185
Total lipid (fat)	g	0.56	2	0
Ash	g	6.61	9	0.62
Carbohydrate, by difference	g	9.57	0	0
Fiber, total dietary	g	1.3	0	0
Sugars, total	g	0.60	0	0
Minerals				
Calcium, Ca	mg	168	6	20.086
Iron, Fe	mg	2.85	6	1.35
Magnesium, Mg	mg	121	3	6.813
Phosphorus, P	mg	42	0	0
Potassium, K	mg	89	0	0
Sodium, Na	mg	233	3	149.706
Zinc, Zn	mg	1.23	5	0.174
Copper, Cu	mg	0.130	8	0.028
Manganese, Mn	mg	0.200	5	0
Selenium, Se	mcg	0.7	0	0
Vitamins				
Vitamin C, total ascorbic acid	mg	3.0	0	0
Thiamin	mg	0.050	2	0
Riboflavin	mg	0.150	2	0
Niacin	mg	0.470	2	0
Pantothenic acid	mg	0.642	0	0
Vitamin B-6	mg	0.002	0	0
Folate, total	mcg	180	0	0
Folic acid	mcg	0	0	0
Folate, food	mcg	180	0	0
Folate, DFE	mcg_DFE	180	0	0

NUTRITIONAL CHART: SEAWEED, KELP, RAW

Choline, total	mg	12.8	0	0
Vitamin B-12	mcg	0.00	0	0
Vitamin B-12, added	mcg	0.00	0	0
Vitamin A, IU	IU	116	0	0
Vitamin A, RAE	mcg_RAE	6	0	0
Retinol	mcg	0	0	0
Vitamin E (alpha-tocopherol)	mg	0.87	0	0
Vitamin E, added	mg	0.00	0	0
Vitamin K (phylloquinone)	mcg	66.0	0	0
Lipids				
Fatty acids, total saturated	g	0.247	0	0
4:0	g	0.000	0	0
6:0	g	0.000	0	0
8:0	g	0.000	0	0
10:0	g	0.000	0	0
12:0	g	0.000	0	0
14:0	g	0.031	0	0
16:0	g	0.110	0	0
18:0	g	0.086	0	0
Fatty acids, total mono unsaturated	g	0.098	0	0
16:1 undifferentiated	g	0.004	0	0
18:1 undifferentiated	g	0.086	0	0
20:1	g	0.000	0	0
22:1 undifferentiated	g	0.000	0	0
Fatty acids, total polyunsaturated	g	0.047	0	0
18:2 undifferentiated	g	0.020	0	0
18:3 undifferentiated	g	0.004	0	0
18:4	g	0.004	0	0
20:4 undifferentiated	g	0.012	0	0
20:5 n-3	g	0.004	0	0
22:5 n-3	g	0.000	0	0
22:6 n-3	g	0.000	0	0
Cholesterol	mg	0	0	0
Amino acids				

NUTRITIONAL CHART: SEAWEED, KELP, RAW

Tryptophan	g	0.048	2	0
Threonine	g	0.055	2	0
Isoleucine	g	0.076	2	0
Leucine	g	0.083	2	0
Lysine	g	0.082	2	0
Methionine	g	0.025	1	0
Cystine	g	0.098	1	0
Phenylalanine	g	0.043	2	0
Tyrosine	g	0.026	1	0
Valine	g	0.072	2	0
Arginine	g	0.065	1	0
Histidine	g	0.024	1	0
Alanine	g	0.122	1	0
Aspartic acid	g	0.125	1	0
Glutamic acid	g	0.268	1	0
Glycine	g	0.100	1	0
Proline	g	0.073	1	0
Serine	g	0.098	1	0
Other				
Alcohol, ethyl	g	0.0	0	0
Caffeine	mg	0	0	0
Carotene, beta	mcg	70	0	0

SEAWEED, KELP, RAW- Scientific Name: *Laminaria spp.*

NDB No: 11445 (Nutrient values and weights are for edible portion)

Source: Nutrient data by UDSA SR20. Each "~" indicates a missing or incomplete value. Percent Daily Values (%DV) are for adults or children aged 4 or older, and are based on 2,000 calorie reference diet. Your daily values may be higher or lower based on your individual needs.

Made in the USA
Lexington, KY
12 October 2014